INTERMITTENT FASTING FOR WOMEN 101

The Ultimate Step-by-Step Guide for Beginners with Delicious Recipes to Lose Weight Fast, Slow Aging, Increase your Energy and Live your Healthiest Lifestyle

Melissa White

By reading this document, the reader agrees that under no circumstances is the author responsible for any losses, direct or indirect, which are incurred as a result of the use of information contained within this document, including, but not limited to, — errors, omissions, or inaccuracies.

TABLE OF CONTENTS

INTRODUCTION

The concept of intermittent fasting means a lot of things to different people, both in meaning and practices. Although this might be the case, intermittent fasting is a diet routine that rotates between short periods of fasting with no food or substantial reduction in calories. It mostly has to do with restricting yourself from eating or cycling between periods of fasting and eating.

There are different ways of observing intermittent fasting. There is a version that advises observing a 24-hour fast once or twice a week. Per week, you're expected to cut off your intake of calories a few days and then spending the rest of the days feeding on regular food. There are other kinds that set limits to your consumption of meals and snacks once you eating window opens. The time to do so usually falls within six and eight hours a day.

To fully grasp the idea of fasting, it is important that we set straight what fasting alone means, something which is not new to us. Fasting involves a stable abstinence from eating food and taking beverages for several hours of the day, mostly twelve hours to one month or more than. It might call for a complete abstinence or a slight reduction in the intake of food and beverages. Fasting as a whole has been used for spiritual purposes, as a mark of tradition, a global ritual for health benefits promoted to influence the body's composition of mass and weight, and also as a tool of political statement across the world.

If fasting is stable, then intermittent fasting is a break between regular meals. It means, for instance, not eating your regular evening meals when you're supposed to have eaten it at the normal time. A good angle of understanding this is this: If you're to skip your evening meal from 8pm in the evening to 8am in the morning the next day, it means you must have observed a 12-hour fast. You can elongate the fasting time to, say, a 15-hour or 16-hour fast if you spent up to 11am or 12pm respectively before having your first meal. You can avoid your meals every day and then feed on two meals when you do so. Your first meal should be taken in the afternoon around 1pm, and then around 8pm of the same day, you can then have the second meal. To observe a 16-hour fast, have your meal the next day at 1pm, which was the precise time you did so yesterday.

You can go as long as several days observing this form of fasting if you choose to do so.

Does it sound strange and dangerous to you that anyone in their sanity would want to fast for 16 hours? When you consider all the great benefits involved in intermittent fasting, you wouldn't think that way at all.

As a woman, intermittent fasting depends heavily on your body and your inclinations. This does not also, in any way, forego your initial aims for engaging in intermittent fasting. A lot of people may readily choose to skip their meals in the morning until dinner time or the next meal.

However, there is something else to remember. Intermittent fasting isn't just about skipping your breakfast or any meal at the time you're supposed to have had it. There's more to it.

Intermittent fasting calls for a total fast for effect. Once you've grown used to this lifestyle, your body automatically readjusts itself such that you no longer eat more than you should when the time comes to do so.

CHAPTER 1
HISTORY OF INTERMITTENT FASTING

What makes intermittent fasting different than any other forms of dieting is that it is not a modern fad; rather it is an age-old technique that has been rediscovered and brought back into the limelight by certain people. It is like Yoga of the world of food.

You will be surprised to learn that people have been fasting since ancient days, perhaps right from the beginning of the human race. If human bodies and evolution are to be considered, eating many meals and snacks throughout the day is neither necessary for survival, nor are they good for health. In fact, an excess of food, like the excess of anything can be extremely harmful to the body. In ancient times, the availability of food was unpredictable and irregular. It was difficult to gather and store food. Seasonal changes too made it difficult to come across food often. For instance, it was easy to get food in summers; however, it became excessively scarce in winters. This phenomenon of fluctuating food and food sources continued until the modern era for everyone except the upper class. In the last century, droughts, famines, wars, diseases, disorders, etc. led to the depletion of food sources. All of these led to starvation and sometimes death as well. It is no wonder that one of those famines is one of the Four Ushers of Apocalypse.

The history of fasting can be roughly divided into three eras - ancient, medieval, and modern. Let us have a look at all three one by one.

Ancient History

The age of scrounging and gathering ended when humans discovered agriculture, perhaps by accident or observation. Once we discovered and developed agriculture, the incidents of famine went down. Agriculture led to the development of societies and culture and religion soon followed. Soon, people all over the world realized that going hungry for a limited period was beneficial for the health of your mind and body. This was then the first instance of periodic fasting. Periodic fasting became a staple of almost all the religions in the world. Forced starvation was replaced by controlled and voluntary fasting as it made people calm, happy, and healthy. It is no wonder that fasting was often called 'detox' 'purification' 'purge' 'ritualistic cleaning' in ancient times. The ancients believed that fasting held the power to clean the body and the soul and that it could help them to please God(s).

Spiritual Fasting

Religious or spiritual fasting still enjoys a strong position in all major religions. Buddha, Christ, and Prophet Mohammad all believed in the power of fasting and advised their followers to fast periodically. It should be noted that fasting as a practice developed intrinsically and independently in varied cultures and religions. This means that people all over realized that fasting had some benefits. Christians follow with Lent; Hindus with various fasts and the Muslims followed Ramadan fasts. Similarly, the Buddhists and Jain came up with certain eating times that they must follow. All of these are types of fasting.

Fasting for Health in the Ancient Times

If we are to consider the history of fasting for health benefits, we should be grateful to Ayurveda and the ancient Greeks. Ayurveda, I.e., the ancient medical science from India called for various forms of fasts and foods for different ailments and general wellbeing. Hippocrates aka the father of Modern Medicine also wrote a lot about fasting and obesity. Obesity was on the rise in the times of Hippocrates in ancient Greece. This was due to the lavish lifestyle and lack of health routines for the royalty. Hippocrates observed the correlation between obesity and early deaths and advised exercise and diet for obese people. The diet he advised included healthy food items and most prominently eating once a day only. After Hippocrates, Plutarch, the great historian, too understood the importance of fasting. Great thinkers such as Plato and Aristotle followed this.

The ancient Greeks believed fasting could improve mental and cognitive abilities and thought it could help them solve problems and puzzles with ease. While this sounds a bit preposterous, try to imagine how bloated and uncomfortable you feel after having a large meal. Meals make you lethargic as your body focuses its energy on the digestive system. You feel excessively sleepy and often doze off after a heavy meal. Some people call this condition a sleep coma. In contrast, if you avoid eating food for some time, you feel far sharper, active, and attuned to the atmosphere. Mind you, this is no accident; it's an evolutionary effect. In the Stone Age, our senses became sharper when food was scarce.

Medieval Times

Even in medieval times, the popularity of fasting did not wane; rather it continued to grow. Paracelsus, a Swiss-German physician who is well known as the father of toxicology, was a proponent of intermittent fasting. He was a firm believer of the theory that anything in excess can prove to be lethal and advised fasting for wellness. One of the founding fathers of the USA, Benjamin Franklin was a proponent of intermittent fasting. A man of many talents, Franklin was a polymath who was well-versed with many arts and sciences. Famous author Mark Twain too was a supporter of fasting for health.

Modern History of Fasting

While the rise of intermittent fasting as a regular diet is a recent phenomenon, fasting, in general, continued its journey from medieval times to modern times. References to fasting can be found as early as the late 1800s. Interestingly fasting developed as a form of entertainment in the late 1800s and early 1900s. The fad died though, thankfully.

Fasting became a staple of medical literature around the early

1900s. Journal of Biological Chemistry defined fasting as a safe and effective way of losing weight and reducing obesity. However, obesity was perhaps the last thing on the minds of people in the early 20th century. The world was changing rapidly, and wars and famines had become commonplace. People were dying for epidemics and starvation all over. With the rise of obesity in the 21st century, fasting once again became popular.

Fasting and Evolution

Fasting was a part of human evolution, and our body and mind are used and perhaps require regular periods of fasts. As most of the citizens of the developed and developing nations have access to ample food regularly, we have almost forgotten about fasting, and it is no wonder that some people look down upon it. Still, intermittent fasting is becoming popular as more and more people see positive results.

Science Behind Intermittent Fasting

While every diet and fitness addition into your life comes with upsides and downsides, intermittent fasting has more pros than cons. If you approach intermittent fasting with an open mind, you'll find that it can help you reach your weight loss goals. In the next part more will be shared about the science behind intermittent fasting and what you can do about your hunger while fasting.

There is plenty of information and research that backs up intermittent fasting. As fasting is not a new thing, extensive research can be found on this topic. Intermittent fasting may soon become a fad, but thankfully it is a fad that is based on science. While much of the research on fasting has been done on animals, the science is still promising.

Fasting is not a new phenomenon. Fasting has been shown in the past to help the body to reset and clear the mind. Interestingly, science goes far beyond that. While there are several different theories as to why intermittent fasting works, one fascinating theory that has been well-researched is that intermittent fasting puts your body's cells under mild stress. When these cells are stressed, they keep adapting and can fight off disease better. Stress is something that often carries a negative connotation.

On the contrary, stress is not inherently a bad thing. When you put your body under stress, positive results can occur. Think of when you exercise hard. You are exhausted and tired, but once your muscles recover, they are stronger. Research has shown that your body's cells respond to intermittent fasting very similar to exercise.

The reason you will lose weight while intermittent fasting can be attributed to a few different causes. For one, it will be much easier to eat fewer calories in the limited eating window. If you are eating on alternate days, during a window period, or skipping certain meals, you will tend to be consuming fewer calories than when you were eating multiple meals throughout the day. Another reason you may lose weight while fasting is because when you stop eating for an extended period, your body goes into its adipose tissue fat cells for energy. Ketones are released into the bloodstream that carries fat, and you end up losing your body fat through your urine.

Research also shows that short-term fasting increases your metabolism speed. Your metabolism is what digests your food. When it works faster, it burns more calories, leading to more weight loss. While many other diets may limit your calorie intake, intermittent fasting does both things. You increase the calories you expend (by boosting your metabolism), and you also decrease the calories you eat. This creates a large calorie deficit. If you exercise on top of intermittent fasting, your calorie deficit becomes larger, and you will lose even more weight.

Intermittent fasting did not become a craze just because of weight loss. Intermittent fasting is popular amongst many already fit individuals because of the other benefits it comes with. One of these benefits is reducing the chance of insulin resistance. Type two diabetes is on the rise. Research says that intermittent fasting leads to a drop in blood sugar levels. Fasting, insulin was seen to drop as much as 20-30% and fasting blood sugar dropped by 3-6%. When you have lower insulin and blood sugar levels, you are at a lower risk for developing insulin resistance, which leads to type two diabetes.

If you are looking for anti-aging benefits, intermittent fasting may be the diet for you, too. Our bodies go through a process called oxidative stress. Oxidative stress leads to aging and many of the chronic diseases that we see on the rise today. Harmful free radicals react with our body's proteins and DNA and damage them which leads to these diseases and aging. However, studies have shown that intermittent fasting increases our body's ability to attack these harmful free radicals. This can help us to combat the effects of aging.

Fasting is also good for the heart. It's no surprise that cardiovascular disease is currently the number one killer in many countries. Intermittent fasting can help stabilize the brain's hormones and brings about better heart health. Fasting can reduce the risk of heart problems with risk factors such as LDL cholesterol, blood triglycerides, blood sugar levels, and inflammation levels lowered. If you have high cholesterol or are on medication for cholesterol and high blood pressure, intermittent fasting could lead to you dropping this medication.

While not proven in humans yet, intermittent fasting has shown impressive benefits in preventing cancer in animal studies. When these animals underwent intermittent fasting, they survived longer and had a reduction in symptoms from their tumors. Cancer is a disease that is not entirely understood and any research showing that this diet can help prevent it should be taken seriously. There was also a study that looked at humans going through chemotherapy. They found that the individuals who followed an intermittent fasting diet had fewer side effects from the chemotherapy. More research will need to be studied to understand fasting's relationship with cancer, but so far it seems to be very positive.

There have many good effects shown throughout research on intermittent fasting but how does it work? How does intermittent fasting cause all these great benefits?

Just as calories from vegetables are better than calories from chocolate cake, the timing of meal consumption can affect how a human body stores it most efficiently. Usually, when we eat something, our metabolism spends hours burning through this food and digesting it. As the stomach digests this food, it will either use the energy or store the energy as fat. Hence, for someone constantly eating throughout the day, the body is going to use the nearest energy source. It is going to burn the calories of what was just eaten instead of the stored energy from body fat. It doesn't need body fat because it is constantly getting a new stream of energy from the food that is being consumed 3 or more times a day. With intermittent fasting, the body is not provided with consistent food at every few hour intervals. Hence, with the body realizing it is not receiving any food, it starts to burn the calories from stored energy, or fat cells. These fat cells become the only energy source available and therefore are being burned from the body.

This can also happen with one workout while practicing intermittent fasting. During the process of fasting and post-workout, the body does not have enough glucose and glycogen to draw from due to a meal skipped. So instead of burning through carbohydrates, where glucose and glycogen often come from, it is forced to look inward for energy. The easiest energy available is the fat stored in adipose tissue. This helps one to lose weight and become leaner. However, intermittent fasting does not stop there. It also aims to make one more sensitive to insulin. When we eat, our body produces insulin. Many individuals are becoming resistant to insulin because of frequent and short eating intervals on top of the high glycemic index food consumed. The more one eats the more insulin that needs to be produced. While insulin is not inherently bad, if the person is not sensitive enough to insulin, he or she will never feel full and keep eating. Fasting changes how we produce and react to insulin. Due to the lesser amount of food consumed, our body is going to release less insulin. The more insulin sensitive one is, the better the body can store the calories consumed. When one breaks fast and starts eating, the body will either use up that energy immediately, store little of it, or it will be converted to glycogen and stored in muscles for use later. Insulin is what is causing many people to gain weight. This insulin resistance is leading to overweight people and many different diseases. With intermittent fasting reducing insulin fluctuations and production, it creates a bunch of other great benefits.

CHAPTER 2
WHAT IS INTERMITTENT FASTING?

Fasting has become a hot topic as of late. The buzz around intermittent fasting, in particular, opened a door for many women who wanted to lose weight but were worried about the heavy commitment of a day-long water-only fast. It's hard to say exactly what intermittent fasting is because there are a variety of ways to go about it. When you do an intermittent fast, you are going back and forth in a regular cycle between fasting and eating normally. I will cover all types of IF (the abbreviation for intermittent fasting) in this book, and you can decide which best suits your stage in life and goals.

Many women have seen real change happen in their health, thanks to IF. You could join them by following the various tips contained here. The first task we have to complete is giving you a broad overview of all things intermittent fasting: what the benefits are, what the science says, what different kinds of intermittent fasting exist, and what foods you should eat when you intermittent fast.

We can start with the health benefits. Women who follow a routine of intermittent fasting feel that they have more energy, burn more fat, and lower their chances of getting diabetes or heart disease. Researchers looking into IF find that its practitioners have higher success rates than people who do extended, interrupted fasts and people who use exercise as their chief method to lose weight. They suggest the success of IF is because it can be woven seamlessly into the participants' lives without their having to change multiple aspects of their normal routines.

Intermittent fasting eliminates the perfectionism that sometimes ruins other weight loss techniques. IF doesn't ask that you constantly pay attention to the number of calories you consume. It doesn't punish you harshly for falling out of it for one day.

We will learn more about the science underlying IF later on but suffice to say that you can earn the positive health effects of autophagy without doing extended fasts. The experiments studying people doing IF consistently demonstrate that they see good results from only doing IF, without doing more demanding fasts such as extended water fasting.

We talked about the study showing that women have more success in losing weight by reducing caloric intake compared to when they pay close attention to what they are eating. This is precisely what IF entails.

I hope that I have at least made you curious about getting these results from IF in your own life — and to do that, you will need to find a way to implement IF in a way that works for you. It's time to answer the question directly: in the simplest terms, what do I have to do to start intermittent fasting today? What is required of me to start seeing these effects on my health?

Because of the nature of IF, you will, unfortunately, have to start tomorrow, not today — unless it is morning right now. Ask yourself how many hours you think you can fast tomorrow. Let's say it is 6 hours. Most people start their fast after lunch and break it for dinner. Keep in mind that you will have to eat lunch relatively early so that you do not have dinner too late. If you have dinner too late, your system will take hours to start up autophagy while you sleep because you will still be digesting food. You should be able to see now why many women find they are able to succeed in losing weight with IF when they were not successful using other methods. What I described in the last paragraph is all that IF amounts to on your end.

Of course, practice is always harder than theory. I will never tell you that intermittent fasting takes no willpower and resistance on your end. Compared to other potential options, though, IF is extremely straightforward. Still, you might have a long way to go to be ready to live by IF. Maybe you still need to be convinced by the number of studies that we will cover proving the health benefits. Maybe you are scientifically minded and need to learn more about autophagy.

You might get inspired when I tell you all the delicious foods you can eat when you intermittent fast to make autophagy even stronger; you might be ready to start after you read about all the different kinds of IF, and you find the one that is perfect for you.

The chapters after this one will explore these topics and more. This one will give you a general idea of all of them so you can keep reading with an informed picture of what you are getting into. You may even choose to check the Table of Contents and read the chapters that interest you the most first. It is your choice. Just be sure to read through all of them at some point, so you don't miss any important knowledge.

Intermittent Fasting: Looking at its Effects on Health More Closely

In few words, IF helps you lose weight using short-term and long-term strategies, by depriving your system of calories so you accumulate less fat in the short term and by detoxifying your cells in the long term through autophagy. The short-term strategy is what tends to draw women in, but the long-term strategy is what makes IF great for your body overall.

This is not the same kind of detox that you may be sick of hearing about online. The autophagy triggered by IF is a detox that has always existed in biology and can simply be jumpstarted naturally by fasting. While a detox like "juicing" will claim to clean out your system, supporters of juice diets have no data to back up this assertion. Meanwhile, autophagy has been studied by scientists and nutritionists for decades now. We know that it works to lose weight. We know that it does so without hurting your body the way that other methods do — not only does it not hurt your body, but it has long-term positive consequences like less inflammation and lower cholesterol.

Every organism on the planet goes through autophagy, so you are not even putting your body through anything strange to get these effects on your health. If you had never heard of the word autophagy before, it would still occur in your body. By learning how to trigger autophagy through intermittent fasting, you are simply learning how to optimize it. Autophagy doesn't involve any strange medicines or foods. Whatever you put into your body; you can still trigger autophagy with IF.

Of course, your diet does affect how powerful your autophagy is, but we will talk about that in a moment. For now, I want to tell you more about the short-term effects of IF. The first we will explore is the enhanced health of your skin. The first layer of skin that you have is called the epidermis. You see your epidermis every day because this is the visible part of your skin. There are layers of skin below it, but you don't see those layers unless you suffer an injury. We will go into more scientific detail on the process of autophagy in the section after this one, but you will need a crash course to understand why autophagy triggered by IF is so good for your skin, and your epidermis in specific.

Both parts of the English word "autophagy" are of Greek origin. "Auto" has the meaning "self" (which you might already know) and "phagy" has the meaning "eat." Put the two together, and you get the fundamental concept of autophagy. Your cells "eat themselves" when they are under acute stress. Unlike you, your cells need energy constantly — even when you are sleeping. They will get it from whatever source they can find. Even when you are not putting food into your body (even when you are fasting), your cells find ways of getting energy. When in this state of stress, their main sources of energy are the following: cell organelles that stopped working, proteins that are no longer being used, and toxins that came from outside your body.

For your first fast, you will notice big changes in your body after only a day. These drastic changes are thanks to autophagy. I guarantee you the first change you will notice is in your skin. It will remind you of when you were younger because of its newfound elasticity and glow. These improvements in your skin are because of autophagy. On an invisible level of your skin pores, your skin cells are cleaning out the toxins described above. On the massive scale of your whole pore, that makes a huge difference. The autophagy results in skin that isn't filled with cellular waste.

The cleaning out of cellular waste isn't the only reason your skin gets better. It's also because you have an increase in the collagen protein in your skin. Collagen is a protein that your skin cells make more of when you are younger. Collagen is the reason the skin of younger people looks the way it is. As you get older, your skin cells make less collagen because they are less effective. This is where autophagy changes everything. Autophagy does two things to make new, young cells: (1) builds them from scratch using the raw materials obtained from eating their own cellular waste or (2) renovates existing cells with new organelles constructed with raw materials obtained from eating their own cellular waste.

Everything should be coming together with intermittent fasting and autophagy now. It all goes like this: you do even a moderate level of fasting that increases your autophagy and then when your skin cells go through autophagy, they make younger cells or make existing cells like younger cells.

The best part is that the improved health of your skin is only the beginning. The main reason everyone who does IF does it is because they want to lose weight. Fasting proves time and time again that it is the best way of doing it. This point has already been driven home, so I will add just one extra point to it: you won't just lose weight, but you will be able to relax about loose skin as well.

The infamous "skin curtain" is the excess skin that people are afraid of getting when they lose weight. It is astonishing how many people say they don't want to lose weight out of fear of loose skin. The good news is that autophagy comes to the rescue on this front. By losing weight through fasting, you cut down on calories and trigger autophagy at the same time. Autophagy's job is to break down poorly performing cells and replace them with new, young cells, or at least replace their organelles with new ones. That's why people who lose weight through fasting are proven to deal with far fewer issues with loose skin. Not only do they have less loose skin to deal with in the beginning, but they are better able to manage what loose skin they do have because of the better health of their skin.

I told you that you would have more energy when you did intermittent fasting, and now it's time to explain the scientific reason why. Autophagy is behind it, as usual. Maybe you have already deduced why by now. The short answer is that the autophagy that IF triggers makes your cells more efficient, and more efficient cells means more energy for you.

As you get older, your cells are less effective than they used to be. They are littered with cellular waste and their cell organs (organelles) are damaged and ineffective in themselves. Autophagy is the remedy to this problem. Autophagy disposes of organelles that aren't performing optimally and disposes of cellular waste and misfolded proteins that are taking up space in your cells without doing anything useful. When all of your cells go through autophagy regularly and take care of these issues, you have more energy because your cells make up all of you, and that makes your system more efficient with energy overall.

Now let's go in more detail on the long-term positive health effects of autophagy triggered through intermittent fasting.

There is research showing that autophagy will fight against tumors, and there is also research showing that it will help them grow — only because cancer cells are cells, too. But although autophagy can work on both sides, the important thing is that autophagy promotes the health of your non-cancerous cells, which will always outnumber your cancerous ones in the early stages. Of course, most people triggering autophagy are doing it to prevent cancer in the early stages and not to stop cancer that is already progressing, so this is all they need. Intermittent fasting has been found to be a powerful tool in combating cancer. While cancer, in general, is still under debate as something that autophagy can prevent altogether, the jury is no longer out for Alzheimer's disease, Parkinson's disease, and Huntington's Disease. We know that these are preventable with autophagy now. Autophagy has been proven to be incredibly effective for matters of the brain.

For long-term problems especially, autophagy is a powerful tool for ensuring the viability and survivability of cells. Scientists did not see autophagy as such a big actor for these diseases until recently. This discovery changes everything scientists thought they knew about the biological process. Excitingly, as I keep telling you, you can trigger autophagy yourself through intermittent fasting.

But cancer is far from the only age-related condition that autophagy can address. Diseases of the mind, heart disease, diseases related to autoimmune failure, and more can be helped with autophagy. While we still aren't sure if autophagy can stop tumors from continuing to grow altogether once they reach a certain size, we know that they can keep the rest of your body around the tumor healthy. This can only be a good thing for fighting cancer, and its why autophagy is useful in preventing all these other diseases too.

In diabetic people, there are clusters of protein built up in their arteries. When they use intermittent fasting to trigger autophagy, scientists can see that these protein clusters are cleared out.

Sometimes books about the newest findings in science with regard to health can be misleading about what the scientific consensus is, but I want this one to be clear about what all scientists agree on. This way, it is as useful and truthful to women as possible.

We know for sure that autophagy is a main player — if not the main player — in fighting against neurodegenerative diseases like Huntington's, Alzheimer's, and Parkinson's. It plays this role by cleaning out the build-ups of proteins that happen in your neurons, leading to clogging and brain dysfunction.

Scientists even agree about what causes these protein buildups in the first place, at this point. As your autophagy occurs in the brain, a special organelle called the autophagosome binds with your lysosome (your cell stomach). In many cases of autophagy, this is the normal way that it occurs. Your autophagosome binds with your lysosome in order to break down the cellular waste.

However, what causes the protein buildups is the abnormally strong bond that the autophagosome has with the lysosome. This strong bond between the autophagosome and the lysosome causes what biologists call a "clogging effect." The clogging effect makes your proteins build up in your neurons, leading to neurodegeneration.

You can read more about the details of this science soon enough, but these are the basics of what causes these diseases. As you can see, autophagy is at the very center of it. If you want to prevent these diseases — as everyone does — you have to trigger autophagy as much as possible, so your cells clean out your proteins.

You might think this sounds counterintuitive since these buildups happen in the first place because of autophagy occurring and the autophagosome binding too tightly with the lysosome. But this abnormal binding is only an issue when your autophagy is occurring at a maintenance level. Scientists who study autophagy say that your autophagy is in "maintenance mode" when it is happening at a low level, just as it always does. You see, autophagy is always happening in your body somewhere, but that does not mean it is happening at a significant level.

Your autophagosome and lysosome can cause the "clogging effect" when your autophagy only happens in maintenance mode and you do not trigger advanced autophagy to clean out the resulting protein buildup. All you have to do to clear out this protein build up is do intermittent fasting, trigger advanced autophagy, and prevent the protein buildup that could cause you to go through neurodegeneration. If you want to know more about the biology of this process or about the link between neurodegenerative diseases and autophagy. For now, we will continue outlining the long-term benefits of using IF to trigger autophagy.

We listed losing weight as a short-term effect, which it is — but it is also a long-term benefit. People who are overweight or obese have higher risk of heart disease, diabetes, and failing autoimmune systems. When you lose weight, you lower your risk of all these problems. Therefore, you should also consider it to have a long-term positive effect on your health.

While this won't apply to every woman's situation, there has also been testing on the effects of autophagy on people going through chemotherapy for cancer. The researchers looked at a group going through therapy without fasting and a group who did intermittent fasting during the chemotherapy.

The group that fasted while going through chemotherapy had significantly lower amounts of dead white blood cells in their systems. If you don't know already, chemotherapy has some negative side effects when it kills cancer cells, and one of them is killing good cells like white blood cells.

White blood cells do a very important job when they are alive, but like every other cell, they become toxic when they die. Unfortunately, chemotherapy tends to kill a lot of white blood cells in the process of killing cancer cells.

That's where autophagy comes in. The patients who fasted during chemotherapy had significantly less dead white blood cells creating toxins in their bodies because intermittent fasting got rid of them. Intermittent fasting led their bodies to seek nutrients from inside the body; there were a lot of dead white blood cells in their body, so autophagy took care of those. As a result, they did not have all these dead cells polluting their bodies.

There is a lot of research about the effect of autophagy triggered by fasting on people with cancer. Another study looked at women with breast cancer who did a fast lasting 12 hours daily. These women did not see their cancer return as often as women who did not fast. This means that not only does autophagy have implications for lessening the side effects of common cancer treatment likes chemotherapy, but it can even lower the chances that your cancer will come back once it goes.

We are still waiting to see if pharmacists can manage to create a medicine that will take advantage of the power of autophagy. There are supplements that claim to trigger autophagy, but none of those claims are substantial at the moment, so your best option is to focus on making autophagy happen through intermittent fasting. But it is possible that, one day, scientists will use their knowledge on autophagy to create a medicine that cures diseases like Alzheimer's and cancer. The possibilities are endless for autophagy.

As far as long-term benefits of autophagy go, it has even been shown to lower the amount of inflammation in your body. When you have less inflammation in your body, your DNA in your cells is far less likely to be damaged. Damaged DNA and high inflammation are big risk factors for diseases like cancer, so these are highly important long-term effects. When parts of your body are inflamed, autophagy does its part by taking care of these damages. Once these damages have been taken care of, you can make new parts that are newer, younger, and less vulnerable to damage. It has even been shown that mice who were bred in a lab who went through autophagy triggered through fasting had lower rates of cancer than rats who did not fast. The ones who did not trigger autophagy had higher rates of cancer.

Your digestive health is surprisingly important to your long-term health outcomes, and autophagy can help in keeping this part of your body healthy as well. It is so important because the parts of your body that control your digestive system are constantly working — they never stop. When they give your digestive system a break by fasting, you are giving it time to stop what it is doing and do repairs. Your tissues in your digestive system have the opportunity to clear out cellular waste and make their systems more efficient at the cellular level.

This makes this system of your body more efficient, all because you are able to trigger autophagy to keep it clean. People often underestimate the importance of their gut health, but it is actually one of the parts of your body you should protect the most. If you are not able to get nutrients with a healthy gut, none of the other systems in your body are able to work the way they should.

We would be remiss to forget about your autoimmune system in the context of autophagy. Your autoimmune system is the way your body attack infections and disease. It fights cancer before it can grow to the size of a tumor. But it isn't only about cancer: your autoimmune system keeps any infection from turning into a disease.

Doctors now say that preventive medicine is the most important kind of medicine, and your autoimmune system is the main player in your body's natural disease preventive mechanism. When you do intermittent fasting, you keep this vital system healthy and prevent age-related disease. This is a good place to start when describing all the good things autophagy can do for your body by simply limiting the window of time that you are eating every day. However, if you want to get the short-term and long-term effects, you have to keep a few things in mind.

First of all, you can't expect to get these results by simply fasting every once in a while. If you eat poorly, drink a lot, smoke, get little sleep, or have any number of habits that are bad for your health, you can't expect to do intermittent fasting and have it repair all the damage you do to your body from these habits. Successfully triggering autophagy with intermittent fasting requires that you are at least somewhat healthy in other areas of your habits as well. Autophagy needs your body to maintain some level of basic health in order to do its job. It can't do that job without your help.

There is not enough space in this book to tell you how to stop all of these bad habits, but I will do our best to consider the lifestyle of the average American woman when helping you get intermittent fasting into your life.

CHAPTER 3
HOW INTERMITTENT FASTING WORK

Although intermittent fasting may seem like an ideal diet plan for those who want to lose their weight or improve their health, you ought to choose the best diet plan for you. You should note that intermittent fasting has some advantages and disadvantages, before getting to know which precautions you should take note of while fasting.

Advantages of Intermittent Fasting

Intermittent fasting has incredible benefits not only to women's body and brain but also to men's. The following are a few of the benefits linked to intermittent starvation:

Altering the functioning of body cells and hormones: Intermittent fasting practiced for a while brings several alterations in your body. For your body to make more fats accessible, it tends to initiate significant cell repair processes and also changes the levels of hormones in your body. The levels of insulin in your body drop, facilitating the breakdown of fats. Growth hormones also increase as the blood levels in them increase a factor that facilitates muscle gaining. The body induces processes such as cellular repairing and removal of any waste materials from the cells.

Lose of weight and belly calories: Intermittent fasting is done to lose weight as you only take in a few meals. Intermittent fasting enhances your metabolic rate, which helps your body burn excess fats such as the belly fats. Studies show that intermittent fasting leads to a 3-8 per cent weight loss if done for around three to twenty-four weeks. Observation shows that within this fasting duration, four to seven per cent of people lost their belly fats, one of the toxic fats in a human's body responsible for various illnesses.

Reduces the resistance of insulin:

Intermittent fasting reduces the insulin levels in your body that, in turn, lowers risks of Type 2 Diabetes, which has been a common illness. The common characteristics of diabetes include high levels of blood sugar in the situation of insulin battle. Thus, intermittent fasting helps in lowering the levels of insulin, which helps in preventing this illness. It also helps protect any possible damages that can affect your kidneys.

Reduction of oxidative constant worry and body inflammation: Intermittent fasting helps reduce stress, which is one of the riskiest ways of fast aging as well as other chronic illnesses. Free radicals are the molecules responsible for reacting with molecules such as DNA and proteins and destroy them. Intermittent fasting, therefore, helps fight body inflammation and destroy any molecules responsible for constant worries.

Heart health: Intermittent fasting is beneficial for your heart's health and prevents you against any heart diseases. Since it regulates sugar levels in your body, intermittent fasting prevents you from high blood pressure, and inflammatory markers, and cholesterol levels hence maintaining the heart health.

Induction of cellular restoration procedures: When you fast, your body initiates the cell's 'waste elimination' procedures that are known as autophagy. Body cells break down and metabolize the dysfunctional proteins that accumulate inside the body cells. Increased waste elimination prevents your body against other illnesses such as Alzheimer's disease, one of the common neurodegenerative disorders with no cure.

Prevention against cancer: After your body eliminates any dysfunctional cells that accumulate over time, your body becomes free from any cancer risks. The uncontrolled development of cells is one of the common characteristics of cancer, and therefore, intermittent fasting facilitates your body's metabolic rate, which helps reduce any possible risks of cancer. Intermittent fasting also reduces several impacts of chemotherapy.

Brain health: Since intermittent fasting is better for your body, then it is best for your brain. Reduction of oxidative stress and various worries is advantageous for your brain fitness. Recurrent fasting increases the development of new nerves, which improves the functioning of your brain. It also helps in increasing brain hormone levels known as the Brain-derived neurotropic factors, which helps fight depression and any other brain-related illnesses. Intermittent fasting also helps fight brain damages caused by stroke.

Extending lifespan: Intermittent fasting can help you live longer due to its ability to control metabolism rates, regulating blood sugar levels, and eliminating any dysfunctional cells within your body.

Disadvantages of Intermittent Fasting

Unfortunately, intermittent fasting has cons too, especially to the females. Studies show that before trying intermittent fasting, you should always contact your physician. The following are the disadvantages associated with intermittent fasting:

It is not risk-free: Intermittent fasting is not advisable to people who are at higher health risks such as those over sixty-five years. People under medical conditions, high fat needs, the diabetic, the underweight, the underage, pregnant, and those breastfeeding cannot undertake intermittent fasting.

You will be hungry: During intermittent fasting, you might have grumbling stomach, especially if you have correctly been observing the correct dietary plans. You should avoid looking at, smelling, or even thinking about food while fasting since this triggers the releasing o gastric acids in your stomach, which then makes you hungry. Engage in some other activities but if you wish to fill your water, drink herbal tea or other drinks free from calories. You may note increased food intake in the non-eating days where you are not limited to any calorie intakes. Intermittent fasting triggers binge food consumption. There could also be cases of cravings, especially after increased levels of cortisol hormone.

Dehydration: Lack of eating may make you forget to take water.

You might fail to take note of the thirst cues when fasting.

Fatigue: Intermittent fasting makes you feel tired, especially if you are trying it for the first time. Your body tends to run short of energy and disrupts your sleep patterns, and this comes along with a feeling of being tired.

Irritability: Since intermittent fasting helps in mood regulation, it can as well regulate your appetite. It leads to being depressed and upset.

Intermittent fasting long-term consequences are not known: Since no one knows whether after losing weight, you will maintain the same for some years, studies claim that no relevant evidence to support the extent of intermittent fasting. You are therefore always advised to talk to your doctor for sound advice on how you should practice intermittent fasting.

There are precautions that you should undertake when practicing intermittent fasting. Fasting has been there since time immemorial, and in some religions, it is considered as a holy practice. Whatever way, you may start practicing intermittent fasting; you should follow its essential tips to avoid any inconveniences. Therefore, you should:

Ensure that your body is fit for fasting. It is by making sure that you are not pregnant, not under any medication, no health complications, not underage, or even diabetic. If you cannot fast, then you can always change to cleaner eating habits such as eating natural foods and eliminate any sugar, rich, or fatty foods from your diet.

Before starting intermittent fasting, you should always try and consult your doctor. Your doctor will give updates about your health concerns and advise whether the step is necessary or not.

Try and make intermittent fasting fit into your lifestyle. You should never fast during the times you are stressed or under excess exertion. It is advisable if you are a newbie in intermittent fasting to try the 5:2 way of fasting whereby you can fast on the first day of the week, then on Thursdays so that you can prepare to take your favorite meals over the weekend.

Before you start intermittent fasting, do not gorge yourself with a 'last supper' but you should instead take healthy meals, lean proteins, and vegetables. Fruits have natural sugar, and including them in your meal could mean a lot. A little amount of starch could make the meal complete, as well. A meal that has all these nutrients will make your body survive the fasting period.

Prepare your household, body, and thoughts before starting intermittent fasting. It means that you should have enough rest and get prepared emotionally. Think about your aim and how to achieve it. Make sure that you hide or keep out of reach any foods that could tempt you during your fasting period.

Stop pretending to be a hero, even when your body is weak. Do not push your body too hard in the name of fasting. There are some of the symptoms that should be of great concern during your fasting time. You should take note of heart shudders, light-headedness, and general feebleness. It requires the use of common sense because you cannot force your body to do what it cannot.

Do not engage in tough exercises; do light ones. Engage in massages as they help have even blood flow in the body parts full of calories, thus reducing cortisol. Do not burn the muscles for energy while fasting.

Always take your vitamins depending on the method of fasting you choose. That acts as a supplement, especially if in liquid form as it eases the process of digestion. They help compensate the vitamins lost while fasting.

Never forget to take a lot of water every fasting day. Your urine should alert you if it is not light in color. If not so, drink desirable amounts of water for proper hydration.

Since you are fasting, it is an obstacle to associating with your friends who are having fun; eating chocolates and drinking wine since you will get tempted to take some. You can indulge in other ways of having fun with your friends. You can pay a visit to the nearest mall, window-shop new clothes or electronics. Avoid grocery stores and any dinner dates. Clear any mouth-watering photos from your gallery.

Avoid getting stressed since stress increases the levels of cortisol, which is responsible for fat storage and muscle breakdown. You can practice yoga, meditating, or having deep breaths. Your body needs enough energy to last you during the fasting period, and so these exercises should be light and not vigorous.

To avoid freaking out, you can always invite your friends to accompany you in doing intermittent fasting. The idea of creating your fasting thread or checking online for any other people doing intermittent fasting can help you master your progress. That is the time that you should focus on mentally cleaning your closet and reflecting on what you are doing.

Avoid 'Victory Binging.' Many people indulge themselves after the fasting period. You should take in a healthy meal and avoid foods that cannot get digested easily. You should take in foods rich in fiber and if you are alcoholic, remember to take care when resuming.

Troubleshooting Problems

What if you do everything and yet there are no visible results. We all have been there at times. It isn't something new or unique to you. But, despite knowing this fact, desperation and disappoint starts engulfing. It is a problem that we all face several times in our lives when we become unsure.

Tackling this problem is crucial and hence learning to troubleshoot the problems is important.

Troubleshooting Problems:

Not Getting Results

This is one of the problems that most people face when they begin any new routine. The fight with obesity is tough, and it has been long. There is a sense of desperation in almost everyone who is trying to lose weight, as most measures prove to be ineffective. So, you become skeptical and unsure.

There is no problem in having doubts, yet trusting the process is also very important. The middle way between both is to set smaller milestones.

However, while you set milestones, do not keep the first milestone very close. You would have to remember that your body would need time to enter into ketosis. It will first have to burn the glycogen stores and then only burning any fat would be possible. Therefore, you must wait very patiently for weight to go down.

All this while, you must follow a healthy diet, observe the fasting time carefully, and increase your activity level. If you do that, you will start witnessing results.

Weight Plateaued

Some people feel that their weight gets plateaued at one level and they stop losing weight any further. There are two aspects to this problem.

First, you stop losing weight, but you still keep losing belly fat. If that is the case, then your progress is still going on, and it is going in the right direction, and there is nothing to worry about.

Second, there is no further progress at all. The first instinct people have in such circumstances is to increase the fasting time or make things tougher. I believe that is not the right approach as intermittent fasting is a long-term approach. Your body only stops losing weight or fat while you are following a healthy lifestyle when it needs to make corrections. Apart from weight, there are several other health factors that need to be taken care off. Even a healthy weight definition differs from person to person. Therefore, jumping on such conclusions would be hasty.

The best resort would be to make some positive changes in your food choices and activity level. Try to increase your exercise. Include more fiber and fat in your diet. Take a diet full of anti-inflammatory foods. These things will help your body in getting healthier.

Always remember, the fat is not a liability for the body, but it is an asset. The body would try to maintain a healthy body fat ratio that it deems necessary for your wellbeing. You only need to keep working sincerely and leave the rest to your body's better sense.

Feeling Dehydrated

This is a problem most people can face. When you begin intermittent fasting, your body starts the cleansing process. It-dumps a lot of water out of the body, and along with with it a lot of minerals also get flushed out. This can make you feel dehydrated and energy drained. The best way to get over this problem is to keep drinking a lot of fluids.

Drinking water is a good way to rehydrate yourself, but only drinking plain water wouldn't be a very wise decision in the beginning. During the cleansing process, you will keep drinking water, and the body would keep flushing it out. There are a lot of toxins that have to be cleared. However, the body, along with water, also keeps losing minerals. You have to prevent this from happening.

You can drink water with a pinch of sea salt. Drinking electrolytes is also a good idea as it also restores the mineral balance. Fresh lime water is another good option in front of you. It helps you in restoring the minerals, and it never gets boring to drink some unsweetened fresh lime water. Besides these, there is no risk of calorie intake too. Hence, you can drink all these things anytime you want.

Braving the Headaches

At the beginning of the intermittent fasting schedule, there will be some negative symptoms like mind headache, lightheadedness, nausea, irritation, and bloating. These are temporary symptoms that arise due to sugar withdrawal or during keto-adaptation. There is no reason for you to worry about them as they would subside pretty fast. However, having unsweetened black tea or coffee can help in alleviating these symptoms.

CHAPTER 4
INTERMITTENT FASTING FOR WOMEN BENEFITS

Numerous studies prove and reiterate the multiple benefits of intermittent fasting leveraged by our ancestors knowingly or unknowingly. Intermittent fasting has positive effects both on your body and mind. When you start your regime, you will notice many good things taking place in your body.

Health Benefits

Maintains healthy blood sugar levels

Carbohydrates from the food we eat are broken down into glucose or sugar in our bloodstream. Insulin transports the glucose from our bloodstream to the cells where it is converted into energy. Diabetes is a condition in which insulin does not function effectively, leading to high levels of sugar in the bloodstream along with multiple symptoms such as frequent urination, thirst, and fatigue.

Studies on intermittent fasting eating patterns have proved that it helps in maintaining blood sugar levels by preventing insulin, sugar spikes and crashes leading to reduced risks of diabetes. Other studies were conducted with participants who had diabetes, and the observations from these studies revealed intermittent fasting not only helped in weight loss and controlled calorie intake but also reduced blood sugar levels.

Studies also proved that individuals on intermittent fasting eating patterns showed a 12% decrease in blood sugar level and a 53% reduction in insulin levels. These figures are reflective of the power of intermittent fasting methods in maintaining healthy blood sugar levels. Lowered insulin levels in the bloodstream prevent build-up which, in turn, increases our insulin-sensitivity allowing the critical hormone to work more efficiently.

Improves Heart Health

Intermittent fasting is proven to have a lot of benefits for heart health by lowering the incidences of certain heart-related risk factors or health markers as they are known in medical terminology.

Studies proved that intermittent fasting reduces unhealthy triglycerides and LDL cholesterol levels and increases healthy HDL cholesterol levels. In some intermittent fasting studies on animals, it was observed that adiponectin protein levels improved. This protein involved in the metabolism of sugar and fat is believed to be useful in the prevention of heart attacks and heart disorders.

Intermittent fasting is also known to balance blood pressure levels, another key risk factor for heart problems. Although many of these studies are animal-based, experts are of the opinion that these benefits could be manifested in humans too.

Reduces Inflammation and Oxidative Stress

Although inflammation is nothing but our body's natural immune response to any kind of injury, chronic inflammation can potentially cause health disorders. Some studies have connected chronic inflammation to cancer, heart disease, obesity, and diabetes.

Studies on people who were following the Ramadan fast showed reduced levels of inflammatory-related risk factors. Nighttime fasts were also linked to lowered levels of inflammatory markers. Alternate-day fasting studies revealed lowered risk factors associated with oxidative stress, another marker directly connected to risks of chronic diseases.

Oxidation is a process that involves free radicals, or unstable molecules, to react with and damage healthy and stable molecules such as proteins and DNA. Multiple studies have revealed the usefulness of intermittent fasting to build our resistance to oxidative stress.

Improves Brain Function and Cognitive Abilities and Reduces Neurodegenerative Risks

Most elements that are good for your body are typically good for the brain too, and so it is with intermittent fasting. Intermittent fasting is shown to improve multiple metabolic features critical for the health of your brain and improved cognitive functions.

These metabolic features that get a boost with intermittent fasting include reduced inflammation, oxidative stress, reduced blood sugar levels, and improved insulin sensitivity. Some animal studies have revealed that intermittent fasting can help in the growth of new nerve cells which could have a direct connection to brain function.

Additionally, intermittent fasting is believed to improve levels of brain-derived neurotrophic factor (BDNF), an important brain hormone. BDNF is a protein which interacts with the nerve cells in the basal forebrain, hippocampus, and cortex; all of which are linked to human cognitive functions such as learning and memory.

BDNF is also known to facilitate the survival and growth of existing neurons as well as stimulating the growth of new neurons. It is also connected to the neuro-synaptic connectivity between neurons. The deficiency of this critical brain hormone is connected to depression and other brain-related mental disorders including cognitive impairment, memory loss, and Alzheimer's. Antidepressants increase the level of BDNF, and so does fasting.

Animal studies have also revealed that intermittent fasting could protect the brain from stroke-related damage. Intermittent fasting studies on animals have also revealed that it could delay the onset or reduce the symptoms of neurodegenerative diseases such as Alzheimer's, Huntington's, and Parkinson's.

Healthy Pancreas and Liver

The pancreas is the organ responsible for the production and release of insulin. As your body becomes sensitive to insulin, the pancreas does not get overworked by overproduction of this critical hormone leading to a healthy pancreas.

Intermittent fasting is also known to make your liver healthy by helping it fight against excessive storage of fat. Intermittent fasting produces proteins responsible for the absorption and storage of fatty acids in the liver, thereby freeing it from having to absorb and hold too much fat.

Improved Sensitivity to Hunger Cues

Leptin, a hormone produced by fat cells, is connected to satiety. It sends signals to you to stop eating when satiated. Leptin levels increase when you feel full and decrease when you feel hungry.

As fat cells produce leptin, obese and overweight individuals typically have high levels of leptin in their body. Excessive leptin potentially leads to leptin resistance thereby making it difficult for your body to read and turn off hunger cues when you are feeling full.

Studies conducted on people who were following intermittent fasting revealed lower levels of leptin during the fasting period. Reduced leptin levels typically translate to improved leptin sensitivity, enabling your body to interpret hunger cues well and prevent overeating.

Intermittent fasting helps in correcting eating disorders by enhancing the body's sensitivity to the various hormones. It helps in reversing binge eating and resetting the natural eating pattern of the human body.

Improves Lifespan

Intermittent fasting studies on animals have revealed its ability to extend lifespan. Many studies on rats gave startling results wherein the rats that were on alternate-day fasting lived 83% longer than those animals which were not on any fast.

Other Healthy Changes in Your Body

Improved Productivity and Energy

When we consume excessive foods, especially processed foods, our minds become dull and our energies are at a low level. On the contrary, studies have proven that on an empty stomach, focus and concentration powers improve significantly.

When you fast, the energies that would have been used to digest the consumed food will be channelized for other more productive work including cell repair and regeneration. Additionally, enhanced cognitive powers (a benefit of intermittent fasting) also help in improving alertness, focus, and mental accuracy.

Fasting makes you feel 'light' which gives you an energy boost. Another reason for this boost of energy is that during a normal eating pattern, our energy source is from carbs and sugars which provide 4 calories per gram. When on a fasting pattern, your body draws energy from fats which give 9 calories per gram, thereby boosting our natural energy levels.

Improved Skin Texture

Oxidative stress from free radicals and chronic inflammation can damage and cause your skin to wrinkle up and form fine lines as well. Intermittent fasting reduces both oxidative stress and inflammation resulting in improved and smooth skin texture.

Intermittent fasting helps clear your skin of acne and pimples, giving it a glowing, vibrant look.

Improved Lean Mass

During any weight loss program, you would typically lose both muscle and fat. Losing fat is great but losing muscle is not. Intermittent fasting speeds up fat metabolism, resulting in more fat loss and insignificant lean mass loss.

Flatter belly

When the body turns to fat for its fuel, it succeeds in breaking down and releasing energy from stubborn belly fat too. Therefore, a sustained effort at intermittent fasting is bound to help you achieve a flatter belly than before.

Improved Motor Skills

Motor abilities such as balance can be affected significantly with aging. There are multiple studies which prove that improved fasting helps in decreasing the effects of motor disabilities associated with aging.

Improved Sleep

Research has proven that intermittent fasting can improve sleeping patterns and can reset your sleeping pattern if it has been disturbed by travel.

Improved Sensitivity to Taste

Getting addicted to excessively sugary, salty, and processed foods is easy. However, the overwhelming tastes from these types of foods lower our taste buds' sensitivity. The taste buds forget how to appreciate and savor wholesome, earthy, and healthy flavors.

After a fasting period, your taste buds are reset to the original natural state, and these grainy and earthy flavors become delicious again. Moreover, as you sustain your fasting efforts, you will notice that you will lessen the amounts of sugars and salts in your food to savor their taste. Even the subtlest of flavors are easily discernible by your sensitive taste buds.

Psychological Benefits

In addition to physical and other health benefits that fasting offers, there is a multitude of psychological benefits you can take advantage of when you choose the intermittent fasting way of staying healthy and fit. Let's explore some of these psychological benefits.

Improved Willpower

Sabotaging behaviors, destructive addictions, and giving in to your desires without a fight are all examples of the opposite of willpower. All these elements slowly but surely ruin your life and relationships. Bad decisions taken because of the lack of willpower will weaken you even further and stunt your growth and development.

If you continue to justify your poor decisions because of your weak willpower, you are only adding fuel to the fire, creating irreparable bad habits for life. Bad habits reflect your inability to control yourself, and if you cannot control yourself, you can hardly control anything else.

Fasting is a natural way of learning to control your responses and reactions to your physical needs and desires. When you fast, you are voluntarily choosing not to eat, even under the pressure of hunger pangs. You are choosing to fast (give up food) to gain something else (health and fitness).

Food is the most basic element of survival and eating when hungry is the fundamental survival instinct. Therefore, when you control this basic survival instinct by choosing not to eat even when you feel hungry, you will find your willpower increasing in strength. You will find the power to control other less fundamental and yet, debilitating bad habits that are ruining your life.

Fasting is the most natural and the most sophisticated form of workout to build your willpower. If you develop the habit of fasting, you will be able to control many other debilitating habits of your life more efficiently. There are medical studies which prove that fasting can dissipate cravings for alcohol, nicotine, caffeine, etc.

So, build and strengthen your willpower by making intermittent fasting a habit in your life.

Improves Self-Confidence

Self-control is the foundation of self-confidence. Confidence is nothing but a reflection of your ability for self-control. So, when you lose self-control, you are effectively sabotaging your self-confidence. The reverse is also true. When you build your self-control, you build and strengthen your self-confidence.

Lack of self-confidence causes plenty of internal conflicts which have the debilitating power of corroding your willpower. These unceasing internal conflicts leave you exhausted and on a perpetual defensive mode resulting in further reduction in self-confidence.

Now, suppose you build your self-control and behave the way you always intended to behave. The results of these intended actions will build your self-confidence as you develop greater trust in your capabilities and strengths. With each success, you will find the power to take on more challenging goals and tasks and eventually build your self-efficacy to such an extent that you are in complete control of your future and destiny.

Fasting is the most effective way to practice self-control and, consequently, build self-confidence. Medical studies have also revealed that fasting improves catecholamines in your body. Catecholamines (for example, dopamine) are believed to be connected to your happiness, confidence, and feel-good emotions and also reduce anxiety and stress levels.

Improved Clarity of Thought

With enhanced brain functioning and cognitive powers, your ability to think clearly will improve. Eating dulls your thoughts and fasting creates clarity. When you fast, your brain and body can catch even subtle signals, and you can see the things going wrong in your life.

While fasting, you can very quickly notice the incongruent elements in your life such as bad habits, poor organization, lack of purpose and intention, and more. This clear perspective is bound to make you take corrective steps.

With improved willpower and self-confidence, you will find the necessary physical and mental strength to overcome challenges and improve the overall quality of your life. Fasting can be a great resetting mode for the psychological aspect of your life.

Improved Emotions

Excessive eating is effectively an emotional dependency. Foods such as processed sugars, caffeine, and trans-fatty acids, and alcohol are all known to over-stimulate our emotions and, therefore, abstaining from eating occasionally helps in stabilizing our emotions.

Fasting can also reset your negative emotion pattern, and you can break free of their harmful effects. Moreover, fasting helps us have a different perceptive of our environment, enhancing our clarity to see what and how things are going wrong in our lives. Such sharp perceptions automatically drive us to reshape our environments for improved quality of life.

The sustained efforts of intermittent fasting can have startling benefits for you. Each one of the benefits mentioned in this chapter is possible. Some of them may manifest faster than others. Patience, perseverance, and commitment are vital elements to leverage nearly all the benefits of intermittent fasting.

CHAPTER 5

INTERMITTENT FASTING 16/8 METHOD

The 16/8 Method is another name for the Lean-Gains Method plan, which is used as a routine targeted explicitly for the removal of body fat and to improve lean muscle mass. One of the most noteworthy benefits of this type of fasting is that it's incredibly flexible so that it will work well if you have a varied schedule. This safe program provides a fasting window of 16 hours, with hours of eating at 8 hours.

How to Easily Follow the 16/8 Diet

A study was performed by the Obesity Society, stating that if you have your dinner before 2:00 p.m., your hunger yearnings will be reduced for the remainder of the day. At the same time, your fat-burning reserves are boosted. During the fasting period, you should only consume food items that have zero calories, including black coffee (a splash of cream is excellent), water, diet soda, and sugar-free gum. The easiest way to attempt this schedule is to stop eating after dinner in the evening and wait 14 hours from there, which means skipping breakfast and picking things up in the early afternoon.

People Who Cannot Fast on the 16/8 Plan

As with other things in your life, intermittent fasting may not be for you. You may need to avoid the restrictions if you are included in these elements:

- People with eating disorder histories

- If you are taking prescription medications, you can have issues taking them on an empty stomach. If you have diabetes, Metformin may cause diarrhea or nausea. Iron supplements may also cause stomach discomfort. Aspirin may also cause an upset stomach or possible ulcers.

- Individuals with diabetes mellitus – type 1 or type 2

- Individuals who experience many times a drop in his/her blood sugar levels

- Underweight people (BMI$\leq$ 18.5), malnourished, or have other known nutrient deficiencies

- Pregnant women will need more nutrition for the unborn child.

- Nursing mothers will require more nutrients for the baby.

- Children under 18 need more nutrients to grow.

Scientific Facts About Intermittent Fasting

Intermittent fasting can change the function of your hormones, genes, and cells.

Myths About Intermittent Fasting

You Don't Need A Good Plan: You must have a well-formulated

plan such as one used with the ketogenic diet and intermittent fasting in this book. Many studies have indicated this is where the dieters go wrong on the concept of losing weight quickly. A well-formulated ketogenic diet will consist of moderate protein and low carbs. That's where many studies cited by critics seem to get it wrong.

Sometimes, it is merely where you have incorrectly calculated your macros. Or, you might make an error when calculating the net carbs. To reach net carbs, which is the number you use to calculate your daily carbohydrates, you take the total amount of carbs minus the fiber counts to come up with net carbs. A well-formulated ketogenic diet will have the majority of fats based on saturated fats.

You do not keep up with the food you consume. You don't have to walk around with a food scale in your hand steadily or be on your Fitness Pal every minute, but you do need to keep up with everything you eat. If you've been stalled out on your fat loss journey and haven't eaten a high-carb and a low-fat diet for a long time, keeping track gives you a guideline to follow. You may not understand precisely what portion control is, but now you should have a better understanding of using it after all of the guidance provided in your new book. Since you're only allotted 30 to 50 grams a day as a guideline, you need to keep track of your fat intake to make sure that it's much higher than your protein and carbohydrate counts.

Everyone has the same carbohydrate needs. When you begin your keto plan, you may not realize how low the carbohydrate content is. A typical ketogenic diet is designed where you will consume 20 to 50 grams of carbs daily. It will depend on factors, including physical activity. It's best to work with a dietitian so you can calculate your nutritional needs. It is also essential to have professional advice because some people have genetic issues with using fat for energy, which can make the diet more difficult or even ineffective for them.

Keto 16/8 Diet Don'ts

Medications could have an effect on my experience with weight loss and the keto diet with fasting techniques:

It's important to inform your doctor about your weight loss program. He/she may prescribe some medicines that make you gain weight. These are a few to question:

Other Possible Medications Causing Weight Gain:

- Antibiotics

- Oral contraceptives

- Blood pressure medications

- Antidepressants

- Epilepsy drugs

- Allergy medicines

Maintain a Calorie Deficit: While this is true for any diet, it is even more true for intermittent fasting since it can be so easy to overeat once you do eat in such a way that it negates any benefits you might have felt. Remember, on average, you need to burn 3,500 calories weekly to lose one pound each week.

CHAPTER 6

INTERMITTENT FASTING 5/2 METHOD

This method has recently become more popular. Even comedian Jimmy Kimmel follows this style of fasting, with great results. While the 14/10 method is about when you eat, the 5:2 method is about what and when you eat. This method means that you'll eat regularly for five days a week, but then have two days where you eat a drastically reduced calorie diet. While most people eat roughly 2,200 calories in a day, while you're on the 5:2 fast, you'll eat your 2,200 calories for five days, but then eat only 500-600 calories on the two fasting days.

The benefits of having the calorie restriction twice per week means that you are more likely to lose weight, even if you overeat slightly on the days when you follow your normal diet. The 5:2 diet hasn't been more heavily researched than many other kinds of intermittent fasting, but what has been researched shows some promising studies about it. While many studies are with animals as subjects, there are a few with human participants too.

In some of the studies, it is believed that the 5:2 method can reduce tumors in breast cancer and help with other physiological issues in the body. It can help improve insulin resistance and prevent cardiovascular disease. While these studies are promising, just keep in mind that many of them revolved around animals. You can find the studies in the reference page at the end of this book, if you would like to do further research.

In general, the 5:2 method can provide you with weight loss that is on par with people who reduce calories every day. However, some people find reducing calories everyday to be very restrictive. Afterall, there's only so much you can eat on a calorie restrictive diet. However, with the 5:2 method you can eat whatever you want for your eating days, and only reduce your calories on your fasting day. While you can eat whatever you want, you should still maintain a well-balanced diet. Eating only junk food won't help with your weight loss goals, if that is the reason you're choosing to fast.

While the 5:2 method can be very beneficial, some people struggle with their first few fast days. After eating 2,000 calories on day one followed by 500 calories on day two, you can feel almost uncontrollably hungry. However, many people say (anecdotally) that the hunger fades if you keep yourself distracted. Also, so long as you follow the fast for a while, you'll soon no longer feel hungry during your fast days. All of this is anecdotal of course, but it is something to consider when choosing to fast with the 5:2 method.

CHAPTER 7

INTERMITTENT FASTING AND

AUTOPHAGY

utophagy is the natural way your body disposes of toxic chemicals in your cells. You can't see it happening without a microscope, but your cells have been going through autophagy for your entire life without you ever noticing. In just the last twenty years, scientists have learned much about the metabolic process of autophagy. Most importantly for our purposes, they have learned more and more about how autophagy's implications for fighting against disease and aging.

The entire foundation of using intermittent fasting for losing weight and getting healthier is our current scientific understanding of autophagy. We know for a fact that autophagy can help us attain better general health and live longer. Autophagy isn't just for losing weight, however — although it does that job better than any other method. It used to be that people went through autophagy quite often. We went through autophagy more back in the days before industrial agriculture because we did not expect to have food all the time.

Nowadays in the industrialized world, most people rarely miss a meal. We always have food around us. But people back in the day did not even have an expectation to eat every single day. Our bodies went through advanced autophagy very regularly because of this. We can even say that our bodies are more built for not eating every day than they are for eating constantly as we do right now.

Our first encounter with autophagy in the world of science was thanks to the French scientist named Christian De Duve. He and a group of biologists took note of a bizarre organelle that they had never seen before; they named it the lysosome.

Before we knew all that we know now about autophagy, scientists thought that the lysosome was simply an organelle made for disposing of garbage. If you think about it, this doesn't even make logical sense, because there is not really such thing as disposing of something. You can change the form of something, but not dispose of it. If the lysosome were really an organelle that just kept breaking things down without recycling those parts, then eventually those tiny waste particles would build-up with nowhere to go.

Now we have an explanation for this problem because of autophagy, and this explanation has important takeaways for doctors, biologists, and anyone who cares about their health.

The Japanese scientist Yoshinori Ohsumi was the first scientist to get deeply interested in the lysosome of yeast cells. 2016 was the year he won the Nobel Prize when he learned that the lysosome was the center of a cellular process called autophagy. His key finding was that our cells never "dispose of" anything — they simply break down cellular waste into raw materials, and then use these materials to build new structures.

Ohsumi has created a new definition of autophagy. He says that autophagy is the way our cells break down waste materials for the purpose of freeing up space, killing harmful foreign toxins, and creating raw materials that can be used for building new cells. When Ohsumi first started, he was the first scientist to really have any interest in this topic. He started a scientific movement around autophagy when his research uncovered all the implications that autophagy has for our bodies. Not only did Ohsumi uncover much of our modern understanding of autophagy, but he was the one who coined the phrase "cell recycling." Cell recycling is what happens once autophagy is finished.

When your cells have cleaned themselves out, they use these raw materials for constructing things that other cells can use. They can also use these raw materials to create new cells if there is enough.

Now we know that autophagy can be considered the most important process for your cells both individually and collectively. Autophagy matters to your cells individually because it keeps them alive as well as possible; it matters collectively because your cells have to work together to be useful to your body as a whole, and autophagy keeps them working together smoothly when the process keeps them repaired and "cleaned out."

You also need to keep in mind the times that you should be eating these foods. The whole purpose of autophagy is lost if you eat during the times you are supposed to fast. That's because consuming anything puts your digestive system at work. When your body digests food, your autophagy stops. You need to really make sure you are not eating at all during these times that you have designated to be your fasting windows.

Even eating 20 calories disrupts autophagy entirely. You may think that eating a banana or a small snack during your fasting window won't change anything, but that isn't true at all. You would be shocked at how much changes in your body when you put food into it. The fact that so much changes is the reason why autophagy is so potent in the first place — because it is recovering from all the times that you were putting food into your body.

But How Does Your Body Know When To Start The Process Of Autophagy?

A signal must be sent to the organs to start breaking down the cells to produce energy. This can be done in many ways. It is not just fasting that can start autophagy in your body. Here are some other ways of losing weight that you can opt for.

Exercise

The more stress you create in the muscles and cells of your body, the more strongly the cellular cleanup phase will be triggered. All the extensive forms of exercise, including jogging, sprinting, weight training and physical training, regulate autophagy by inducing stress in the body. When the body is highly worked up, it needs energy that it gains by burning up the cellular waste.

Cold Showers

Yes, cold showers can also invoke healthy autophagy inside you. Studies have shown that people who swim during the winter exhibit higher levels of cell repair and recycling. Therefore, taking cold showers regularly can help you lose weight and stay healthy.

Steam Bath

Subjecting yourself to high temperatures through saunas and steam baths generates heat stress inside you. This heat results in the destruction and recycling of cancerous as well as damaged cells.

A trip to a spa can be good for relaxing, rejuvenating, losing weight and staying preventing diseases. Besides, exposing yourself to strong heat also helps to cure depression by naturally releasing heat shock proteins.

Intermittent Fasting

There are indicators in your body that activate or cease certain processes. The hormonal levels are one of them. When you begin intermittent fasting, you deprive the cells of essential nutrients. This activates the hormone glucagon in the body. This hormone works in opposition to insulin. While insulin increases blood sugar levels, glucagon brings them down to maintain the balance. The two hormones are like the ends of a see-saw.

When you are fasting, insulin levels go down, and, as a result, glucagon levels go up. This rise triggers autophagy. Your body gets the message that it is time to break down the stored fats in the body cells increase the insulin levels again.

Antioxidants

Though antioxidants do not directly invoke the process of autophagy in your body, they have been known to indirectly work towards it. Foods rich in antioxidants support the process when you are fasting, which in turn ensures that you undergo a healthy and balanced autophagy process.

Is There Something That Can Stop Autophagy?

There are factors that can stop your autophagy process. The major one is the mTOR. It stops the autophagy in your body when there are enough nutrients in the cells. It is highly sensitive and eating as little as 50 calories can increase the level of mTOR.

If you consume fats, it might not raise your insulin levels, and it might keep the mTOR levels suppressed. But high amounts of ketones and fats would break your fast.

Here is a list of things that you can take to keep your insulin levels low and let your body continue the waste removal process of your cells.

Green Tea

Coconut Oil

MCT Oil

Ginger compounds

Galangal

Reishi mushroom extracts

Black coffee

Apple cider vinegar

All these items can help to boost autophagy in your body.

Is It Just For Weight Loss?

Absolutely not. When the cells renew themselves by burning up the waste inside them, they do more than decrease your weight. Clean and healthy cells decrease the risk of developing diseases. Many forms of cancer, neurodegenerative diseases like Alzheimer's and Parkinson's, and metabolic and autoimmune diseases can be prevented through autophagy.

It helps fight infectious diseases and regulates inflammation. It has also been associated with fighting depression and schizophrenia. Fasting-induced autophagy is very helpful in keeping you healthy and preventing medical conditions. It is always good to get rid of the waste around and inside you. A clean environment is healthy and keeps you from getting sick.

Here is a list of major benefits of autophagy, both inside and outside of a body cell.

Increases metabolism

Decreases oxidative stress

Increases genomic stability that prevents cancer

Eliminates waste from the body

Increases neuroendocrine homeostasis

Decreases inflammation

Increases lifespan

Eliminates aging cells

Improves muscle performance

Does Autophagy Help Women? How?

The ghrelin or the hunger hormone increases more quickly in women than in men. Women start feeling hungry again quickly after having a meal. Their bodies start craving food much faster and, therefore, are under more stress to look for energy sources. The cleansing of their body cells makes them less immune to catching diseases and helps them to develop a stronger immune system.

Does Autophagy Have Anti-Aging Effects Too?

Consider a real-life example. Assume that you have two cars, X and Y. You are somehow biased towards car X, and so you take much better care of it. You wash it every day, get it serviced every few months, and refuel the tank. But car Y does not see many bright days. It is just a backup option for you for the days X is out for servicing or repairs. You do not get its tank refueled, it stays covered in dirt and has been for just one servicing in years.

Now, which car do you think would last longer? Obviously, car X. When you pay attention to health and get the repairs done on time, faults and damages do not pile up. Your car X would stay as good as new even after years of driving, but car Y would start causing trouble very soon.

The same thing happens with the cells in your body. When the non-functional components and cellular waste keeps sitting inside the cell, it degrades your health and makes you look older. But when they keep recycling and renewing, it shows on your skin. Rejuvenated and youthful cells make your skin softer and healthier.

Autophagy is like a cellular garbage disposal system. Newer cells wash away the dead and unhealthy ones. This leads to increased elimination of aging cells. Autophagy slows down the aging mechanism of your body that makes you look younger and healthier for a long time.

How Does Your Body Renew Itself Through Autophagy?

Small things matter, and when it comes to aging, small things are the only ones that matter. Cells are what keep you healthy and sick. They store energy, carry oxygen and do everything for your body. And they are the ones that keep you from aging on the inside and outside.

Let us understand how this works. The cells in your body are continuously at work, so they experience a lot of wear and tear. The over-used cells eventually stop working, thus becoming useless. When this happens, the production of new and healthy cells is also discouraged by the useless ones.

These used up cells are known as senescent cells. A senescent cell is a living cell, but its functioning does not contribute to maintaining person's health. And while they do not contribute to anything, they do not let new cells to get formed in the body either. Over the years, the senescent cells keep accumulating in the body. They perform just baseline functions, stop the creation of new cells and promote inflammation. The worst part for women is that they speed up the aging of the nearby cells.

Autophagy clears away the damaged cells, thus making way for the youthful cells to appear. You stay young, healthy and energetic for a long period. Therefore, working towards burning up the waste in your body cells is a great thing for you to do.

Developing healthy habits in your life is a good way to live. No one likes an untidy home; while a shining home with new furniture is loved by all, including the ones who live there. Autophagy is a way to throw away all the old things from home and make space for refreshing new things.

CHAPTER 8

FOOD TO EAT DURING

INTERMITTENT FASTING

We can distinguish 4 different categories for different types of drinks and effects they have on fasting:

- 0 kcal liquid foods that enhance the effects of fasting. Do not be afraid, during fasting periods when you will not have to touch food and therefore you will not consume meals, you will have the opportunity to drink non-caloric drinks, the important thing is that they are not sweetened. In this category we have foods such as vinegar, coffee, green tea, black tea, multivitamin supplements (which I recommend taking with vegetables and not on an empty stomach), WATER. Stimulants, such as caffeine, which mediates the production of norepinephrine which mobilizes glucose stores and increasing the ADP / ATP ratio in turn activates AMPK / PPAR which is enough to let us know that they are all events that enhance the mobilization of acids fats and catabolic processes involved in fasting. As for water, which is often not considered too much, drinking a good quantity of water at one time causes a rise in pressure mediated by the norepinephrine, which reconnected to what has been said about stimulants makes us guess that it has a very important.

- Caloric liquid foods that potentiate the effects of fasting.

Among the foods that we can consider non-zero calories, we certainly find famous BCAAs (even if they are powdered, they must be dissolved in water and therefore we consider them liquid), branched amino acids, even if they supply calories to our body, for a direct effect on the limitation of muscle catabolism (they are gluconeogenesis, they are used in place of the amino acids obtained from the destruction of muscle to produce glucose) they bring benefits for fasting. Another "surprise" food in this category is coconut oil, although it is a fat and therefore very caloric, it does not interrupt carbohydrate fasting, it activates the metabolic pathways that promote lipid oxidation, but being mainly composed of acids Medium chain fats (MCTs) will be very quickly, and likely directed to the mitochondria rather than being accumulated as fat. Other similar foods are ghee or clarified butter, largely composed of MCT fat.

- 0 kcal liquid foods that block the effects of fasting (or have no effect on it). There is not much to say about this category of liquids, because it should not even exist since there are practically no calorie foods that block the fast, but only foods that have no effect on it, although not interrupting it, we could think of sweeteners, but from several researches recently published, it has been noted that they have an (indirect) influence on the release of insulin, mediated by the perception of "sweet taste". Obviously a few drops in coffee or tea will not block the fast, but it will not have positive effects either, they are "neutral". An example of drinks are "zero" sodas, which if you follow Martin Berkhan, you know you can take in quantity.

• Caloric liquid foods that block the effects of fasting. Practically the most intuitive category; sugary drinks and liquid foods that bring more than 50 kcal per 100g, if you like a drop of milk in coffee, it will not be the one to block it (provided it is a drop and not milk coffee). For solid foods we have a greater limitation, practically there are foods that block fasting (calories) and foods that enhance their effects (calorie or limited calorie <50 kcal per 100g).

• Fasting foods (calories). All known and intuitive foods, cereals, sweets, dairy products, oils etc etc., in short, all categories of foods that are excluded from fasting (using a little common sense you can easily guess). Foods that enhance its effects (calorie or limited calories <50 kcal per 100g): It is an interesting category, since we find very interesting foods, such as meat, for those who practice a PSMF (Protein Spared Modified Fast) it is practically a fast in which they only take proteins to limit muscle catabolism and spices; Among these we have cinnamon, black pepper, chili pepper, turmeric. They are all spices that act on the catabolism factors (for example, the chili pepper slightly increases the metabolism, making sure that the calories ingested are less than those needed to digest it, on an empty stomach it is a BOMB to enhance its effects).

Now that you know how fasting is "created", you can well try experimenting with combinations of the various foods that will make it much more effective (and pleasant, like fasting coffee for example). An example is that of the famous "Bulletproof coffee",

MCT fats such as coconut oil or ghee (clarified butter) dissolved in hot coffee (or blended together), it may seem crap but I assure you it is a unique goodness, the foam that forms is a pleasure. But also combinations like mint and cinnamon coffee, or mint and vanilla tea, are all tastes that we Westerners are not used to and can seem strong or disgusting; instead in the Far East it has been used for centuries, if in fact you are looking for some 0 kcal recipe with coffee or tea, you will be amazed at how simple it is to enjoy these drinks in countless different (and above all good) ways, I recommend you try Turkish coffee, and I assure you that it will become a ritual to remain on an empty stomach just to savor its full taste!

As for the intermittent fasting supplement, practically all supplements at 0 kcal or that involve less than 50 kcal per 100g are allowed (it is an office value, it is not a magic rule, it is used to establish a range). Multivitamins are also fine, but I recommend taking them with food as soon as the fast is broken since their absorption is greater when combined with vitamins with high biological availability (such as those found in vegetables). More of this goes to isotonic drinks, there is no problem as long as the TOTAL calories of the drink that are under the fateful 50 kcal, be sure to check the value of kcal you take per serving.

CHAPTER 9
PROS AND CONS OF INTERMITTENT FASTING FOR WOMEN

Intermittent fasting has its good and bad side. In this , we'll be going through some of the magnificent benefits of intermittent fasting and its attending downsides. However, it is important to state beforehand that the moment you decide to go into intermittent fasting, make sure you do it wholly "clean."

A clean fast in itself can only happen when it involves only water, tea and coffee without the interruption of fat and other sweeteners. In essence, no calories! I realize that staying off from your favorite ice-cream, coffee and sugar might be one of the most difficult things to for you to do in this life. But, remember, one of the aims of intermitting fasting in the first place is to restrict calorie intake and inhibit your body from triggering production of insulin so as to burn fats. Try to get used to it. The end benefit is all worth the sacrifice.

It is believed that our body cells, hormones, and other vital genes readapt themselves so as to work well during the time we deny the body of regular food. For instance, our growth hormone radically increases when we fast.

Apart from the above, a clean fast is believed to have a positive and massive influence in our aging process. Diseases such as heart diseases, cancer, Alzheimer's diseases and diabetes, all of which can weak the heart and fasten the aging processes can be hindered through a clean intermittent fasting.

The Good Side

Although researchers and health experts have not yet fully understood or satisfactorily studied the benefits of intermitting fasting, its metabolic switches and stress resistance of our cells cannot be overemphasized. Below are some of the good sides of intermittent fasting that women can take advantage of:

- Intermittent Fasting Fights Cancer

Photo credit: Drink Nature's Water

Numerous studies, (notably that of Moreschi and Rous, done a century ago) conducted in animals have demonstrated that by restricting calorie intake daily, alternate-day fasting diminishes and suppresses both spontaneous and induced tumors respectively as the subject rodents age, and increases how sensitive they are to chemotherapy and irradiation. What does this mean for humans? It means that intermitting fasting can create the favorable condition to weaken cancer cells from metabolizing, hinder them from growing and make them disposed to treatment.

- Intermittent Fasting Delays Alzheimer's and Parkinson's Diseases

It is widely known that extreme energy consumption can readily expose you to stroke. Diet control patterns such as the alternative-day fasting can defer the arrival and advancement of Alzheimer's and Parkinson's diseases. Intermittent fasting motivates stress resistance through various mechanisms to help prevent seizures.

- By reducing weight, intermittent fasting can help mitigate the symptoms of

asthma in people who are obese. Its ability to reduce inflammation can also be helpful for fighting rheumatoid arthritis

- Intermittent Fasting Improves Growth Hormone

Intermittent fasting can help boost our growth hormone, thereby strengthening our muscles and bones.

- Intermittent Fasting Improves Cardiovascular Health

Perhaps this is also another reason why people are heavily drawn to intermittent fasting. Studies have shown that IF improves cardiovascular health, including blood pressure, heart rate, and the level of cholesterols in our bodies.

- Intermittent Fasting Is Easier; Dieting Is Harder

Not a lot of people are fully able to stick to a diet plan for a long period of their life. They find it extremely complicated and expensive. Within a short time, you might possibly find them making a U-turn to the "wrong" food that they were hitherto used to. Others might simply fail to follow the diet completely. This is not the case with intermittent fasting, which seems to be simplifying and easy enough to be applied to our eating schedules.

Most obese people find it hard to change their diet, even though they're fully aware that the type of food they consume or binge on is probably responsible for their obesity. Intermittent fasting doesn't seek to change, entirely, these foods, but rather creates a routine for such women to adopt so as to cut down on their calorie intake, so as to burn fat. A lot of people can easily adopt this eating routine than changing their diet completely.

- Intermittent Fasting Increases Longevity

By now, you'll be thinking that if intermittent fasting increases the human life span, everyone, from children to adults, will be into it. After all, even you would love to live a long and fulfilled healthy life. But few people will deliberately starve themselves, even if they're aware it's for their own benefits.

Scientists have for long established that by restricting calorie intake, intermittent fasting has a noteworthy effect on aging and lifespan. It does this by reducing stress, lowering insulin levels, and enhancing autophagy (meaning, "Self-devouring"), the body's ability to sanitize damaged cells so as to generate new and healthier cells.

Photo credit: Dr. Jockers

Studies in intermittent fasting favor the alternate day fasting as the fasting plan that leads to a longer lifespan. This is because of its rotation between zero calories, while feeding on herbal tea, black coffee, broth and water.

Perhaps this is the best time to intermittent fasting if you wish to have a longer and healthy lifespan.

- Intermittent Fasting Easy Life For The Busy People

For women who live a very busy life and have little time to fix breakfast every morning, intermittent fasting is your deal. On your fasting days, you can simply grab that glass of water and your day is made. What this reduces is the stress of planning a meal, cooking and making way for a better but simpler eating schedule. This is a huge additional simplicity to your life. Single and working parents will find this more practically beneficial. It saves your money and time!

The Bad Side

It is highly possible to lose some weight of by restricting your calorie intake and burning fat. You can even enjoy some of the most discussed advantages of intermittent fasting. Yet, there are a lot of reasons why intermittent fasting might be bad for you and why you should perhaps avoid it altogether especially when the fasting seems to be extreme for your health.

Photo credit: The Weight Loss

- Intermittent Is Bad For Those With Eating Disorder

Here, you might have probably thought of bulimia nervosa. If you did, you're absolutely right! The dangers of intermittent fasting on people susceptible to a disorder in their eating habit are remarkable. Through the years, there has been a lot of (some tragic and fatal) reports about models who stay off meals completely for some time so as to achieve the "perfect" body shape. I strongly advise women who have one eating disorder to stay away from intermittent fasting or anything associated with fasting.

• Intermittent Fasting Has Negative Effect On Sugar Control In Women And People With Diabetes

Intermittent fasting has been shown to have a negative impact on blood sugar control in women. This will naturally contribute to abnormalities in their menstrual cycle of most women, and by so doing, decrease their chances of giving birth. For this basic reason, some experts have completely advised women to stay away from intermitting fasting.

On the other hand, women who are diabetic have mal-absorption should also not intermittent fast. This is dangerous for them as it can, again, lead to a reduction in blood sugar level. When this happens, the medication process of the diabetic patient is hampered.

• Intermittent Fasting Has Negative Effect On Women In Their Reproductive Stages

Women who are pregnant or breastfeeding need not go into intermitting fasting. According to healthcare experts, intermittent fasting (especially the Warrior Diet plan) will not only be disadvantages to them as a mother but will also harm the baby, as it can lead to inadequate intake of nutrients such as minerals, vitamins and fiber.

- Intermittent Fasting May Lead To Tiredness More Often Than Usual

Most women who have intermittent fasted have reported their body feeling too tired more than usual. The reason for this is that the body has little access to energy than it used to. Health experts have advised either stopping the fast or to curb their tiredness by having a regular and health sleep and doing little work when the body is in a fasted state.

- Intermittent Fasting Increases Food Cravings

Because intermittent fasting can boost our cortisol, the body's stress hormone, this means an increase in food cravings. A lot of women tend to overeat and binge on food once their eating window opens. At the end of the day, they consume more carb/fat/calories more than they should, making them gain more weight and rendering the initial fasting futile.

- Intermittent Fasting Initiates Mood Swings And Depression

A lot of women reported having mood swings and depression while intermittent fasting. This is because their anxiety and depression neurotransmitters (dopamine and serotonin) have been affected when they decided to regulate their appetite and intake of nutrients during the fast. As a result, they feel easily ill-tempered happy especially when their body is in the fasted state.

- Some people who intermittent fast might not feed on enough nutrients when their eating window opens.

This will possibly deny them of fiber and increase their risk of getting cancer. It might also affect their digestion and immunity against diseases.

CHAPTER 10
BEST RECIPES

Amish Cauliflower-Broccoli Salad

Serving Size: 7

Nutritional Counts per Serving:

- Net Carbohydrates: 3 grams

- Calories: 324

- Protein: 7 grams

- Fats: 32 grams

Ingredients Needed for Preparation:

The Salad:

- Broccoli florets (8 oz.)

- Cauliflower florets (8 oz.)

- Red bell pepper (half of 1/about 2 oz.)

- Cheddar cheese (4 oz.)

- Cooked bacon (.33 lb.)

- Green/purple onion (2 tbsp.)

The Dressing:

- Mayonnaise (.75 cup)

- Full-fat Greek yogurt/sour cream (.75 cup)

- Freshly squeezed lemon juice (1 tbsp.)

- Low-carb powdered sugar - ex. erythritol (2 tbsp.)

How to Prepare:

1. Dice and fry the bacon for about six minutes using medium heat. Drain it on paper towels.

2. Chop the vegetables into a large bowl. Prepare the dressing. Cover the fixings if you are not going to serve immediately.

3. When you're ready to eat, toss everything together and serve.

Chicken Salad With Feta & Kiwi

Serving Size: 2

Nutritional Counts per Serving:

- Net Carbohydrates: 13 grams

- Calories: 314

- Protein: 28 grams

- Fats: 15 grams

Ingredients Needed for Preparation:

- Fig balsamic vinegar (1 tbsp.)

- Kiwis (2)

- Extra-virgin olive oil (1 tbsp.)

- Salt (1 pinch)

- Mixed field greens (4 cups)

- Chopped grilled chicken breast (1 cup - about 5 oz.)

- Feta cheese (.33 cup)

How to Prepare:

1. Chop the chicken and crumble the feta.

2. Whisk the balsamic vinegar, oil, and salt.

3. Add the greens and chicken breast.

4. Peel and cut the kiwi into halves. Dice into 1-inch wedges and add to the salad with the crumbled feta.

5. Toss well to combine.

Chopped Greek Salad

Serving Size: 2

Nutritional Counts per Serving:

- Net Carbohydrates: 2 grams

- Calories: 202

- Protein: 4 grams

- Fats: 19 grams

Ingredients Needed for Preparation:

- Chopped romaine (2 cups)

- Halved grape tomatoes (.5 cup)

- Kalamata black olives (.25 cup)

- Crumbled feta cheese (.25 cup)

- Vinaigrette dressing (2 tbsp.)

- Olive oil (1 tbsp.)

- Black pepper & Pink salt (to taste)

How to Prepare:

1. Toss the salad together using the lettuce as a base.

2. Spritz it using a drizzle of oil and vinegar.

3. Serve in two salad dishes.

Easy Red Cabbage Salad - Instant Pot

Serving Size: 4

Nutritional Counts per Serving:

- Net Carbohydrates: 0.2 grams

- Calories: 131

- Protein: 3 grams

- Fats: 3 grams

Ingredients Needed for Preparation:

- Shredded red cabbage (2 cups)

- Pepper and salt (as desired)

- Coconut sugar (.5 tsp.)

- Red wine vinegar (2 tsp.)

- Coconut oil (1 tbsp.)

- Chopped onion (.25 cup)

How to Prepare:

1.   Place the steamer basket in the Instant Pot and add the red cabbage.

2.   Lock the top. Set the timer for one to two minutes. Quick-release the pressure, and remove the basket.

3.   Rinse the cabbage under cold water and arrange in four portions.

4.   Add the fixings, toss, and serve.

Egg Salad

Serving Size: 4

Nutritional Counts per Serving:

- Net Carbohydrates: 1.4 grams

- Calories: 305

- Protein: 8.7 grams

- Fats: 29 grams

Ingredients Needed for Preparation:

- Hard-boiled eggs (6)

- Curry Powder (1 tsp.)

- Full-fat Mayonnaise (.5 cup)

How to Prepare:

1. Prepare the boiled eggs by adding them into a saucepan. Pour in cold water.

2. Turn the burner on.

3. Once the water begins to boil, set a timer for seven minutes. Pour out hot water when done.

4. Prepare a cold-water bath and submerge the hot eggs into it to stop the cooking process.

5. When cooled, peel and chop the eggs into small bits.

6. Combine the mayo, eggs, and curry powder.

7. Serve with a portion of chopped fresh parsley.

Shrimp Avocado Salad With Tomatoes & Feta

Serving Size: 2

Nutritional Counts per Serving:

- Net Carbohydrates: 6.5 grams

- Calories: 430

- Protein: 24 grams

- Fats: 33 grams

Ingredients Needed for Preparation:

- Shrimp (8 oz.)

- Large avocado (1 diced)

- Beefsteak tomato (1 small)

- Feta cheese (.33 cup)

- Lemon juice (1 tbsp.)

- Cilantro/parsley (.33 cup)

- Olive oil (1 tbsp.)

- Melted salted butter (2 tbsp.)

- Freshly cracked black pepper & salt (.25 tsp. each)

How to Prepare:

1. Devein the shrimp, peel, and pat dry. Dice and drain the tomato, chop the parsley, and crumble the feta.

2. Melt the butter and toss the shrimp in a bowl until well-coated.

3. Warm a pan using the med-high heat setting until hot.

4. Toss the shrimp into the pan in a single layer, searing until it starts to become pink around the edges (1 min.). Flip and cook until the shrimp are cooked through (30 sec. approx.).

5. Transfer the shrimp to a plate to cool.

6. Add all other fixings into a large mixing bowl (diced tomato, diced avocado, lemon juice, olive oil, feta cheese, cilantro, pepper, and salt). Toss to mix.

7. Toss it and serve.

Steak Salad Specialty

Serving Size: 2

Nutritional Counts per Serving:

- Net Carbohydrates: 1.5 grams

- Calories: 403

- Protein: 1.5 grams

- Fats: 33 grams

Ingredients Needed for Preparation:

- Ribeye steak (1- 8 oz.)

- Green salad mix (2 cups)

- Steakhouse seasoning (1 tbsp.)

- Olive oil (1 tbsp.)

- Wine vinegar (1 tsp.)

- Pepper and salt (as desired)

How to Prepare:

1.   Use the steak seasoning to prepare the steak and cook to your liking.

2.   Wait for it to cool while you toss the salad fixings with a dusting of pepper and salt.

3.   Drizzle with oil and toss again.

4.   Slice the steak into bite-sized strips.

5.   Arrange the salad on two serving dishes and sprinkle the steak bits on top.

6.   Serve using your favorite dressing if desired - but count the carbs.

Thai Pork Salad

Serving Size: 2

Nutritional Counts per Serving:

- Net Carbohydrates: 5.2 grams

- Calories: 461

- Protein: 29 grams

- Fats: 33 grams

Ingredients Needed for Preparation:

The Sauce:

- Juice & zest of lime (1 lime)

- Chopped cilantro (2 tbsp.)

- Five Spice (1 tsp.)

- Fish sauce (1 tsp.)

- Red pepper flakes (.25 tsp.)

- Rice wine vinegar (1 tbsp. + 1 tsp.)

- Mango extract (.5 tsp.)

- Tomato paste (2 tbsp.)

- Soy sauce (2 tbsp + 2 tsp.)

- Red curry paste (1 tsp.)

- Liquid stevia (10 drops)

The Salad:

- Romaine lettuce (2 cups)

- Pulled pork (10 oz.)

- Medium chopped red bell pepper (.25 of 1)

- Chopped cilantro (.25 cup)

How to Prepare:

1. Zest half of the lime and chop the cilantro.

2. Mix all of the sauce fixings.

3. Blend the barbecue sauce components and set aside.

4. Pull the pork apart and make the salad. Pour glaze over the pork with a bit of the sauce.

Tuna Salad & Chives

Serving Size: 4

Nutritional Counts per Serving:

- Net Carbohydrates: 1 gram

- Calories: 235

- Protein: 20 grams

- Fats: 18 grams

Ingredients Needed for Preparation:

- Tuna in olive oil (15 oz.)

- Mayonnaise (6 tbsp.)

- Chives (2 tbsp.)

- Pepper (.25 tsp.)

- Salt (as desired)

How to Prepare:

1. Drain the tuna and finely chop the chives.

2. Add all of the fixings except the lettuce into a mixing bowl.

3. Toss well.

4. Enjoy as-is or spoon into romaine lettuce leaves.

CHAPTER 11
COMMON MISTAKES TO AVOID

With a growing amount of people in the world fighting to get healthier, it is no huge surprise there prevailing trends of eating fewer carbohydrates that are popularized through the overriding press.

As signaled from the WHO, approximately 52 percent of the entire population is either obese or corpulent. A high number of those individuals have tried to get fit in any event earlier or later in their own lives, and a few have tried different items with outrageous eating of fewer carbohydrates followed by the fad absorption of fewer calories.

For instance, as the study seems, an outrageous weight reduction diet is not only ineffectual as a very long-haul arrangement, but it very well might be unbelievably harming for your wellbeing.

Outstanding eating of less junk food prompts muscle wasting

Outstanding weight-loss abstinence from food, for the most part, comprise serious calorie restriction with the purpose of shedding a great deal of weight in the shortest amount of period possible. While those ingestion regimens will automatically prompt unbelievable weight reduction within the first barely few weeks, then you need to bear in mind that you risked losing muscle tissue until you discover the chance to shed weight.

As indicated by medicinal experts, eccentric abstaining from excess food consumption will initially prompt water weight loss, at the point of muscular decay, as well as fat hardship. Scientist G.L. Thorpe has explained this quite some time back, expressing that our body does not especially absorb fat when we eat less. It instead, squanders all the body tissues, such as the bones and muscles.

Muscle wasting interrupts your digestion.

The motivation behind why your system aims muscle tissue when you're starving yourself is because it aims to safeguard vitality when nutrition is insufficient. To explain this further -- your system requires additional energy in order to maintain muscle tissue than it will, in order to care for fat.

When there is a lack of energy from nutrition as in cases of absurd eating of junk food, your body will attempt to evacuate among the human body's most noteworthy energy shoppers -- the muscles.

This will occur no matter if you're doing weight reduction clinics you might believe help reconstruct more muscle. Be as it may, the terrible news does not end there.

Recall that lost mass prompts a lower basal metabolic rate, and a reduced metabolic rate inspires you to have more weight reduction. These realities explain why such a high number of people go through the jo-jo effect after an outrageous eating pattern.

A study spread in the Journals of Gerontology found that the calorie restriction decreases vitality expenditure. What this means is that being on a remarkably low-carb diet can prompt more slow digestion which makes future weight-loss problematic if not certainly impossible.

Moreover, slims down which are low in carbs are often restrictive and everything considered, unfit to tackle your body's problems for basic nutritional supplements. Therefore, being on the condition, an 800-calorie diet plan is most likely going to prompt nutritional supplement lack that can damage your wellbeing.

A concentrate that has been dispersed at the Journal of the International Society of Sports Nutrition scrutinized the pervasiveness of micronutrient inadequacies in widespread slims down, and the results were striking.

The evaluation discovered a restrictive weight reduction diet known as the best lifestyle diet fulfilled just 55 percent of daily micronutrient requirements while the exceptionally famous South beach diet fulfilled just 22 percent of their day daily prerequisites for micronutrients. Other negative outcomes are fewer carbohydrates, as well as restrictive weight reduction programs, include osteoporosis, obesity, discouragement, kidney stones, and in extreme instances scurvy if the eating regimen is insufficient in nutrient C.

The best way to get in shape right?

For one thing, you need to bear in mind that successful weight loss consistently goes forward bit by a little bit. This means changing to some wise dieting propensity which is possible to pursue for a substantial amount of time to come as practicing a week per week assumption.

You should additionally consume fewer calories than you personally, as a guideline reach for weight loss to happen. As indicated by means of an examination distributed previously from the Journal of Research in Medical Sciences, devouring fewer calories would be the ideal weight reduction program, especially when combined with low-GI and moderate fat intake. Just make sure that you reduce your calorie entrance by 300-500 calories as indicated by Harvard Health Publications.

For example, if your typical eating regimen comprises of 2500 calories, then begin eating 2200 calories. Your body will put aside the attempt to modify in accordance with this discreet caloric shortfall, yet earlier or later, you can shed a few calories.

Just make sure you don't eat everywhere under 1200 on the off possibility that you're a woman or below 1500 on the off probability that you're a guy to steer clear of micronutrient lacks. Various items to help you with becoming thinner include discovering daily weight-loss inspiration pointers to help prop you up and assessing your health along with your primary care doctor to assess whether fundamental wellbeing requirements are slowing down your weight loss.

Diets do not do the job, yet superior dieting does

Instead of following prevailing fad diet drifts which you see being advanced with lean renowned men and women, nutritionists would advise that you pursue decent dieting.

By switching to smart dieting instead of a low-carb diet that does not work, you will have the choice to shed weight slowly and address your body's problems for essential nutrients.

At this stage, as soon as your body is solid, and your penis is well-supported, you're certain to experience effective long drag weight loss. Another motive behind this is really that intelligent dieting is a good deal easier to stick to over the long haul when compared with unthinkable and restrictive eating regimens.

As per a passing dispersed in the Journal of Food and Nutrition, switching to smart dieting involves creating an enormous way of lifestyle changes, focusing on nutrition quality, and correcting your own nutrients.

A similar section documents the health benefits of fantastic dieting that include the diminished threat of cardiovascular disease, diabetes, malignancy and of course, a better body structure.

Easily Disregard Immediate Weight Loss

You may hear reports of people losing a huge amount of burden by following inconceivable eating regimens. These reports are standard elements of boosting attempts for weight reduction products and abstaining from excess food consumption novels which are conceivably hindering health. Sticking to shown actualities is your principal way possible to get fit efficiently and safely.

Weight reduction requires that you cut down on your calories bit by bit without undermining your health. Additionally, it includes regular exercise to enlarge energy use and to fabricate more muscular tissue.

What is the best diet to get audio weight loss?

Get any eating regular publication and it'll profess to maintain each of the answers to efficiently losing all the weight that you want --and keeping it off. Some propose the secret is to consume less and exercise; others that reduce fat is the ideal thing to do, but others endorse eliminating carbs. Overall, what could be a fantastic idea for you to take?

The fact of the matter is that there isn't anyone size fits all" response for endless sound weight loss. What works for one person might not work for you, because our bodies respond distinctively to different nourishments, contingent upon hereditary attributes as well as other health facets. To find the strategy for weight loss that's right for you may probably need substantial investment and need commitment, dedication, and some experimentation with numerous nourishments and diets.

Even though a couple of men and women respond well to tallying calories or relative restrictive methods, others respond better to get more chances in organizing their get-healthy plans. Being allowed to only maintain a strategic space from singed nourishments or cut back on refined carbohydrates can place them up for advancement. Do not get too disheartened if an eating regimen that worked for one more individual does not do the job for you. In addition, don't pummel yourself whether an eating regimen that you stay with proves unreasonably prohibitive. Invariably, an eating regimen is right for you if it is one you're able to remain with for some time.

Maintain in your mind: while there is no easy remedy to losing weight, there is a lot of steps that you can take to develop a more favorable institution with nourishment, restrain passionate causes to gorging, and achieve a good weight.

Two notable weight-loss systems

1. Cut calories

A few experts accept that efficiently coping with your weight boils down to some simple requirement: If you consume fewer calories than you eat, you get slimmer. Sounds easy, is not that so? At that stage, why is shedding fat so challenging?

• Weight misfortune is certifiably not a straight event after some time. At that stage, once you cut calories, you might shed weight for the very first few weeks, for example, and then something changes. You consume a comparable number of calories; nevertheless, you lose less weight or no fat anyway. That's about the grounds that if you get healthier you are losing water and slim tissue equally as fat; then your digestion alleviates back, along with your own body changes in various ways. Along those lines, in order to keep losing weight weekly, you need to keep cutting off calories.

• A calorie is not always a calorie. The stunt for continuing weight reduction would be to ditch the nourishments which are pressed with carbs but do not cause you to feel complete (like snacks) and supplant them with nourishments which shirt you off without even being piled with calories (such as vegetables).

• a lot of us don't generally consume only to meet hunger. We likewise visit nutrition for relaxation or to calm stress --that can quickly crash any weight reduction program.

2. Cut carbohydrates

An alternative way of review weight reduction modulates the problem as none of devouring such a high number of calories, but rather the way your system amasses fat following to expending sugars--especially the task of the hormone insulin. At the stage when you consume a dinner, then starches in the nutrition enter your circulatory system as sugar. In order to maintain your sugar levels under wraps, then your body regularly consumes this off sugar before it absorbs fat out of a feast.

Maintaining a fantastic wellness

Everybody needs to be strong; however, not a lot of jobs to go the extra mile and adopt a solid propensity on a regular assumption. Whatever the instance, with much more mindfulness towards a healthy and sound means of life, folks increasingly are going in the path of it. The way to maintaining good wellbeing is the combination of numerous elements like regular exercise, excellent eating routine, stress the plank, work-life balance, audio relations, higher assurance, and that is just the tip of this iceberg. Nothing could be substituted for another. In case you're looking for some vital guidelines on the most skillful process to maintain up great health, measure along these lines.

1. Stay hydrated

How to maintain up great health? It is as simple as drinking heaps of water and fluids to keep yourself hydrated regularly. Drinking water generally during this time is essential because we keep losing water out of our own body as urine and sweat. Water does some major capacities, as an instance; flushing germs from your liver, assisting absorption, distributing nutritional supplements and oxygen into the cells, preventing stoppage and maintaining up the electrolyte (sodium) equilibrium.

2. Eat lots of fruits and vegetables

The body demands a constant inflow of minerals and nutrients. An eating regimen rich in leafy foods ensures that your body receives each of the supplements needed. All leafy foods have their own effect on providing different minerals and nutrients. Contain a whole lot of splendid and deep-hued veggies and organic products such as apples, red berries, purple berries, and lush greens since they are wealthy in cancer prevention agents that fight illness-causing free radicals. You prepare a few interesting plates of mixed greens, or perhaps make a yummy organic merchandise chaat or blend them into thick smoothies.

3. Do not limit your meals

Every supper has its own impact. Afterward, skirting among those 3 important dinners of this day may have a negative impact. Your cerebrum and body need fuel to operate. Your brain wants a stockpile of sugar and a lack of it can cause you to get torpid. Skipping suppers can make your digestion down, and this may prompt weight gain or make it more challenging to get healthier. At the stage when you bypass dishes, your body turns on the 'endurance style', which basically implies it succeeds for much more nutrition than anticipated, which finally contributes to pigging out.

4. Prevent fatty, processed foods

The fresher, the better. Affordable food and ready or bundled nutrition often follow various additives and additional substances to enlarge rack live. Furthermore, they may hide substantial levels of sodium and sugar which may construct the threat of life infections like diabetes, hypertension, circulatory stress, heftiness, and the sky is the limit from there. Handled nourishments also have 'satisfying' quality that suggests that for their succulent, sweet or zesty flavor, your head starts thinking about them as remunerating nourishments that arouses superfluous yearnings.

5. Contain more lean meats, low-fat dairy products, and whole grains for your diet

The way to maintain good wellbeing is to get a decent eating regimen with meals grown on the floor. You want a decent mix of milk, milk products, meat, legumes, and vegetables. Select low-fat milk, yogurt, cheddar, lean beef, fish (cut on reading beef), darker rice, millets and oats to get much more favorable outcomes. With respect to grains, whole grains tend to be better. Processed bread and grains such as Maida and white rice saturated in nutritional supplements. Whole grains are piled with fiber and nutritional supplements which keep you full and satisfied; It also comprises of stock Health Practitioner and Macrobiotic Nutritionist Shilpa Arora. The type of starches you eat is important. A huge part of our starches should be low levels which suggest that they should not result in rapid spikes on your sugar levels and provide moderate birth of energy." Whole grains, dals, rajma and vegetables - these are phenomenal wellsprings of unpredictable and very low GI sugars.

CHAPTER 12
HOW TO GET STARTED

At this point, you likely know which intermittent fasting strategy you're going to employ or which ones you're going to try deciding between since there truly are so many options, so it's time to start thinking of how to put your plan into action. While intermittent fasting can seem, to some, much less daunting than an entire diet change, it is just as intense as becoming vegan from being a meat-eater for others. That being said, no matter which camp you fall into, you'll likely need a few pointers for the adjustment period.

The gist of this is to give you the information you need to make the transition into your first (or next) intermittent fast as easy and painless as it can be. You'll be provided with tips to help establish a new routine as well as informational tidbits of what to expect, what to do and what not to do, what to look out for and, for worst-case scenario moments, when to quit.

Before the is finished, you will also be guided through common mistakes in the transition to intermittent fast. The hope is that you'll then be able to avoid such instances in your own experience as you decide how and when to move forward with IF yourself. You'll also be exposed to ways to "protect" against potential hiccups in the plan. Simply put, the more forethought, the better; the more you're mentally and emotionally ready for, the more successful your adventure with intermittent fasting will be overall. Let's make our way into getting started!

Transitional Tips

When you're about to begin your process of intermittent fasting, you'll need to have a few tricks up your sleeve to make the transition as painless as possible, and that's what this section is all about. First of all, make sure you do have some sort of method planned. Pick that plan and stick with it, at least for the first week. Next, do any extra research you may need to do, considering your body type and any diseases or disorders that you may have. This extra bit of research may be game-changing for you, in terms of making sure your transition into IF has no disruptions or toxic effects for your body type. If it's necessary at this point, check with your doctor to ensure that you're on the right track and that the method you've chosen poses no harm to you.

Something else you can do before start IF, is to look at your diet ahead of time and adjust things to be a little easier. As I mentioned before, a diet composed of primarily processed foods may pose complications for the individual during the detoxification period. As you can, start to replace processed foods, with whole foods (fruits, vegetables, grains, nuts, seeds, etc.) that support your health and healing. Additionally, as you plan which method you'll undertake, you can go into more detail and make sure your feasting is packed with the right nutrients between fast periods. Calculate the calories you'll need for each fast, the macronutrients you'll need to refuel, and the training you anticipate you'll be able to handle. The more forethought, the better.

When it comes to that first day of getting started in the intermittent fast lifestyle, the following pieces of advice will help to make things flow with ease. First of all, on the evening before, don't eat a late dinner, and don't eat after dinner. Make sure to have lots of drinks on hand for the fasting process ahead. Healthy and IF-safe drinks are listed above. Imagine that night before that you're beginning your fast at sundown or after that early dinner. Then, when you go to sleep and wake up in the morning, you've already done almost 12 hours of fasting. At that point, delay your breakfast the next morning, and you can easily achieve 12 hours if not 14 of fasting right off the bat.

During this waiting period, have as many IF-safe drinks as needed, and then, when the eating window comes (if you choose a method that involves an eating window or at least if you try this day-1 transition guide), engage in eating, but don't snack too much. The following days, whether they involve eating windows or not, try to cut out snacks more often to help your body adjust. Other things you can do before and during your transition to IF include skipping breakfasts habitually or simply delaying them, having earlier dinners, or substituting snacks for smoothies.

Help for Routine-Setting

After the first few days, you may need a little help getting the routine affirmed and established, and the following pieces of advice are attuned to help with that exact problem. To assist in routine-setting, remember to keep things slow and simple, especially at the beginning of your process. Don't push yourself too hard and keep your expectations for the fast (and on yourself) realistic and grounded.

It could be that you've tried to start with a method that's too disruptive of your standard routine. It's much more productive to transition into something that's a somewhat "logical" extension of your daily activities.

What to Expect

When you begin intermittent fasting, there are several things you should expect from your experience, regardless of whether they're helpful or not. The points below will walk you through those details to prepare you for what's to come.

First of all, mornings may be completely different for you. You will likely find that your mornings become filled with energy or completely lethargic, depending on whether you were a morning or night person beforehand. Furthermore, you may experience your worst hunger pangs during the morning time, but this element is also affected by whether you're a morning or night person. Finally, coffee will become your best friend, if it's not already. Mornings may be the most serious times of fasting for you, and even if they're not fasting periods, you're still going to need that infamous morning juice (coffee, or at least something caffeinated that similarly kick-starts metabolism) to get you through the day as it is now, with less food in it.

Certain things will increase. During your initial transition period into intermittent fasting, your abilities to plan and organize are liable to massively and noticeably increase. You might find that scheduling your fast into your week feels impossible before you begin, but after the first few days, it will become more second-nature to organize and think in this way. Additionally, you will almost certainly become more mindful of the world around you, of your internal feelings, and of how food truly affects you. As one final note, recall all the potential benefits of intermittent fasting. Remind yourself of what you're working to grow in yourself, and you're sure to be propelled through the hard times.

Other things will decrease. The most common goal of intermittent fasting is to lose weight (yay!), and that will almost assuredly happen for every IF practitioner. That weight is bound to decrease with the appropriate application of intermittent fasting and healthy diet, given your body type and physical needs. Furthermore, you may lose sleep, at least during the first two weeks' detoxification period, which is detailed more in the next paragraph. Although sleep may be difficult, it will settle back into a normal pattern, and if you always have troubles with sleep, you might even find that you have the easiest, most restful sleep of your life while you're intermittently fasting.

During a period of the first two or so weeks, you will definitely go through a detoxification period. You will get stinky, moody, cranky, and tired. You will feel weird bursts of energy and then nothing at all. If you're working out as you practice intermittent fasting, you might find that your workouts during the first two weeks are especially exhausting or unproductive. You might have an emotional moment or two, but after these first two weeks, those powerful side-effects should go away, for they're all a part of the detox associated with the transition. You have to get through the rough patch to reap the rewards, however, so stick with the process and fight through those crunchy, harsh times. You'll be thankful you pushed through, no matter how smelly you may get.

Finally, your relationship with food will become entirely different. It may take a couple of days — it may even take the entire detox period to get it right to settle into eating the right amount during your eating windows. At first, you might have trouble with either eating too much or not enough when it's time to eat, but you will be urged to work through any food dependency issues by this process regardless of how often and how much you eat. During times of fast, one can't help but consider with new eyes how food, hunger, and hangry feelings affect one's relationship with others and the world.

What to Do/What Not to Do

When it comes down to it, knowing concisely what to do and what not to do will be the informational backbone to your success with intermittent fasting.

What to do includes:

- Start slow

- Track your progress

- Live normally, otherwise

o Especially in times of fast, work and play are especially distracting when you're hungry!

- Help to suppress hunger with drinks like mineral water and with gum

- Keep tabs on your hormonal health

o As a woman, it is especially important that you perform this work to troubleshoot IF in your life.

- Focus on fats when you eat (without making fat consumption your main goal)

On the other hand, what not to do includes:

- Don't start too hard and fast

o Ease into it!

- Don't give up after just a week

o This is a big no-no unless you display warning signs and worst-case-scenario markers.

- Don't diet too fiercely

- Don't work out too much

- Don't continue to intermittently fast even after you display warning signs

- Don't constantly eat during the eating windows

o Don't forget that your body still needs breaks in eating to digest!

What to Lookout For

As you engage with intermittent fasting, there may be warning signs that your body is not benefitting from the process at hand. You'll have to be very keen and conscious of these warning signs, for if they appear, alterations will need to be made if your success and health are the goals (as they should be!). Overall, look out for warning signs like constant headaches, tiredness without the ability to sleep, dizziness, lightheadedness, or constant sleeping. While some of these elements can be signals that adjustments in the process are all that's needed, if you had any of these problems before trying IF and they've gotten worse as you continued with IF, you may have reached a quitting point.

Something else to look out for includes those general hunger pangs, but as we've discussed before, just make sure to ride those urges out like waves, for they surely will pass. Check in with yourself mentally and emotionally as you proceed with intermittent fasting, too, for your knowledge of yourself will be the most helpful aspect of making sure that your process is healthy for you. If you notice that your personality starts to align with those problematic traits, try scaling down the intensity of your fast, or you could also try processing those personality traits and rescaling them to be appropriate and more health-oriented. The process of intermittent fasting is one that can be easily abused and twisted into something that's unhealthy, but the better you know yourself, and the more you seek growth in this effort, the better off you'll be when it comes to IF.

When to Quit

Since you're female, you are a bit more likely to experience worst-case-scenario intermittent fasting moments than a male would be, but when you do come up against these scenarios, do not doubt that it is truly time for you to stop. Pushing beyond this point means your life stands at risk, and no fitness regime is worth that price. Do not take these worst-case-scenario warnings lightly.

Worst-case-scenario warnings include:

- Burning in the pit of your stomach

o   This sensation is a likely sign of gastritis or something even worse.

- Vomiting even when you've hardly eaten

o   You could have gastric irritation, an imbalance of electrolytes, or something more dangerous.

- Fainting

o   This issue is especially worrisome if it becomes habitual.

- Feeling a pain in your stomach or chest

- Experiencing diarrhea

o   Diarrhea is troubling because can contribute to dehydration and imbalance of electrolytes if not noticed and fixed in time.

- Worrying period symptoms

such as: complete loss of period, excessive bleeding, or spotting when you're not supposed to be

CHAPTER 13
THE CONCEPT OF CHEAT DAYS

Cheat days are the escape routes that people have devised in order to make the torture of any routine bearable. This concept is very effective in diets and calorie-restrictive regimes. However, it pushes the weight loss efforts far back. It is also a fact that once you get into the habit of taking cheat days, the number of such days keeps on increasing. Things soon spiral out of control and become unmanageable.

The concept of cheat days doesn't hold much ground when it comes to intermittent fasting. The reason is, intermittent fasting never puts very hard boundaries that need to be jumped. If you want to eat anything and you are still in your eating window, you can eat it right away. If your eating window is over, you can always eat it the next day. There is no ground for harboring long temptations. Therefore, there is no real need for cheat days.

The people following regular routines like the 16:8 protocol may want to take a day off when they can eat for the whole day. In that case, they can choose to eat the whole day. However, there are certain problems with that:

❖ Eating in an unscheduled manner will trip your hunger clock the next day

❖ Eating certain foods loaded with sweets will lead to cravings.

Resisting them becomes difficult

❖   Your digestion system may also get disturbed

But, if you still want to have the day without rules, you can also have it. Terming it a cheat day will make it more convenient. I believe that it shouldn't become an escape route.

Some experts also believe that when you keep following intermittent fasting for a very long period, the results get slow. I beg to differ here, it isn't the results getting slow, but the need of your body to shed more weight gets low. As you would reach anywhere near a healthy weight, your body would resist losing weight as it wants to remain healthy. However, when you start indulging yourself, you quickly gain weight and hence gain losing it becomes simple. It is simply a matter of looking at things. The important things should be the amount you weigh on the scale but the way you feel internally.

If you feel that following a certain lifestyle is making you feel healthier, you must stick to that plan and not try to make too many changes.

Devising Your Plan

When it comes to intermittent fasting, all the protocols mentioned in the book are simply guidelines. They would act as directive principles where you can make changes to them as per your convenience.

The important thing is to devise your plan, and here 'personal' is the keyword. It is very important for the long-term success of the efforts.

Every individual has a unique body structure. Although we all have a similar organ structure and functioning, yet every individual's response to various stresses is different. Some people may easily withstand hunger for 24 hours without flinching. There are certain people who forget having their meals. However, there are countless of those who have food running at the back of their mind all the time. The way a person would depend on the stresses would depend entirely on that person's unique physical needs and hormonal response.

Therefore, one solution fits all wouldn't work when it comes to intermittent fasting too. You would have to test yourself for a reasonable limit up to which you can withstand fasting. Forcing yourself too hard wouldn't be a very prudent decision.

Women should keep this fact in mind, especially. They have a very sensitive hormonal system which is closely related to starvation triggers. They must never force themselves to extreme hunger as this can have an adverse impact on their fertility, mood, libido, mental and emotional well-being. The best way is to do things in moderation and take your body towards longer fasting in a slow and steady way. They must give their body a chance to adapt to the hunger periods.

There are some points that will help you in devising your own plan:

✓ Always start with the easiest fasting plan.

✓ Before exposing yourself to long periods of fasting, you must eliminate the habit of snacking

✓ If you want to fast without having food cravings and hunger pangs, you must make changes in your food choices

✓ Eliminating sugar and high carb food will help you in eliminating food cravings. These are addictive

✓ Having heavy meals would help you in feeling satiety for long. You wouldn't feel the need to have snacks or meals frequently

✓ Always give yourself at least a month of time at every new plan. This is the time your body needs to get adapted to any fasting schedule

✓ Never choose a fasting plan that's too hard for you. It should always be a little tough but always bearable

✓ You don't have to go by the clock. You can break your fast an hour earlier if you are feeling very hungry

✓ However, you should always try to remain in the fasted state as long as you are not feeling hungry

✓ Don't eat simply because it is time for you to eat

✓ Once ketosis starts in the body, your energy needs you diminish considerably as your body would have unlocked immense energy stored in the form of fat

✓   You must give your body the time to burn fat. Frequent eating without feeling hungry would come in the way of burning fat

✓   Make healthy changes to your diet

✓   Do not count calories but pick healthy options

✓   100 calories from broccoli and 100 calories from pancake are not the same for your body

✓   You body values the nutrients and not the calories

✓   There is no system in the body to count calories it is a misconception

✓   You must start eating healthy food

✓   Eat foods rich in fiber, macro, and micronutrients

✓   Eliminate all kinds of carbonated drinks, soda, beer, alcohol, juices of any kind. These things give you empty calories

✓   Eating fruits is good. Drinking a smoothie which has the pulp is also fine. Drinking juice without pulp is unhealthy. It will spike your blood sugar and not give your digestive system anything to work upon. The same goes for any kind of drink other than water or fresh lime.

✓   Drink plenty of fluids like water, unsweetened fresh lime, electrolytes as your body would lose a lot of water during the cleansing process

✓	Lower fluid intake can lead to the formation of stones

✓	Do the exercise as much as possible

✓	Even if high-intensity exercise is not possible, at least for a walk daily

✓	Live a healthy lifestyle and your fat would burn much faster than you have anticipated

In the end, always choose your intermittent fasting plan as per your requirement.

If you want to lose weight fast:

You must choose shorter fasts like 16:8 protocol or Crescendo fasting

If you want to bulk muscles:

You can choose the warrior fasts or the 20:4 fasting protocol

If you want to lose weight and also get in a healthy shape:

You can choose the OMAD routine or 23:1 intermittent fasting plan. Eat-Stop-Eat or alternate-day fasting protocol also give great results.

If you want to get a healthy body and cleanse it:

You must choose the longer fasts as they can start autophagy rapidly.

You can choose the duration of the fast as per your tolerance and repeat them at an interval of 15-30 days. However, you must always follow them with caution. Going for a longer fast without practice can be difficult.

Keep these things in mind and devise a plan for you that works. Remember, don't go for perfection. The human body is perfect in many terms, and hence you need to be careful. The body would achieve perfection on its own. You need to make small adjustments that suit your body, and that would work great.

CONCLUSION

By eating in a way that follows your body's natural rhythms and needs, you maximize its ability to function healthily. This supports your body with everything from weight loss and muscle gain to balancing hormones and blood sugar levels. There are many different benefits that you stand to gain when you monitor not only what you eat, but when.

Perhaps one of the best parts of intermittent fasting is that this unique diet does not require you to give up on anything that you truly enjoy eating. Instead, you simply change when you eat and enjoy less healthy food choices in moderation. Of course, if you prefer to combine intermittent fasting with another diet, such as the ketogenic diet, then you will have adjusted food requirements. However, the intermittent fasting diet itself does not require you to adjust your food intake to meet any specific needs.

After you have read this book, it is important that you go read this book! If you are going to go ahead and adopt the intermittent fasting diet as well, this book is going to massively support you in doing so. That way, you can understand the benefits of intermittent fasting, as well as how you can embrace both of them to maximize your health benefits.

You do not want to find yourself taking on a new diet only to have frustrating and challenging symptoms such as headaches, fatigue, and stomach aches. This will make the transition painful and, likely, unsustainable as well. Shocking your body in this way is not healthy or helpful. Instead, take it easy and move at a pace that you can reasonably handle. Remember, this is a complete lifestyle change so you can take your time. As long as you are consistently moving forward towards your goal, consider it a success.

It is also important that you take the time to regularly monitor your symptoms and pay attention to your needs. Listen to your body and what it is telling you, as this will support you in really embracing the diet in the most powerful way possible. You do not want to find yourself struggling to succeed because you have made it too challenging for yourself. Going slower and learning to truly listen to your needs now will make your long-term goals far more achievable and sustainable.